The Next Fifty Years

A GUIDE FOR WOMEN AT MIDLIFE AND BEYOND

Pamela D. Blair, Ph.D.

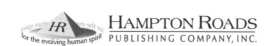

HAMPTON ROADS
PUBLISHING COMPANY, INC.

Cover design by Jane Hagaman
Cover digital imagery © PunchStock/Corbis. All rights reserved.

Hampton Roads Publishing Company, Inc.
1125 Stoney Ridge Road
Charlottesville, VA 22902

434-296-2772
fax: 434-296-5096
e-mail: hrpc@hrpub.com
www.hrpub.com

If you are unable to order this book from your local
bookseller, you may order directly from the publisher.
Call 1-800-766-8009, toll-free.

Library of Congress Cataloging-in-Publication Data

Blair, Pamela D.
  The next fifty years : a guide for women at mid-life and beyond/
Pamela D. Blair.
       p. cm.
  Summary: "Offers women both beyond and approaching fifty encouragement
and practical advice on re-envisioning their lives for the road ahead. Includes
a group study guide and space to journal"--Provided by publisher.
  Includes bibliographical references.
  ISBN 1-57174-439-8 (8x10 tp : alk. paper)
  1. Middle aged women. 2. Aging--Psychological aspects. 3. Women--Conduct
of life. 4. Self-esteem in women. I. Title.
  HQ1059.4.B58 2005
  646.7'0084'4--dc22
                          2005013153

ISBN 10: 1-57174-439-8
ISBN 13: 978-1-57174-439-5
10 9 8 7 6 5 4 3 2
Printed on acid-free paper in the United States

This book is dedicated to my Swedish grandmother,

Agda Matilda Janssen Smith,

and to my mother, LeEsta Davis.

Table of Contents

Acknowledgements xi
Introduction xiii
How to Use This Book xix

Part I

1: Thoughts, Cultural Attitudes, and Myths about Women Aging 3

When They Were Our Age • Myths to Not Live By • Living in the Present •
Changing Tempo • Being Vulnerable • Aging Can Be Fun? • Accepting Change •
Age Grief • Ages and Stages • Aging Is Another Country • An Attitude of
Gratitude • An Attitude of Solitude • Birthdays • Saying What I Mean • The
Decision • Waiting

Part II

2: Our Self-Image 31

Becoming Invisible • You Don't Look Like a Grandma! • Who Is That Old
Woman? • Sagging Faces and Liver Spots • High Maintenance • Feeling Young
Inside • Old Bodies, New Again • Proud of Our Wrinkles • Looking Good • *Now*
Who Am I? • Strong in a Youth-Obsessed World

3: Our Minds 49

Your Brain Is a Muscle • Senior Moments • Mind/Body Connection • Losing
Things • Is It Menopause or Mental Pause? • Memory, What Memory? •
Continued Learning • Brain Growth

4: Our Emotions 62

Bad Moods • Is It Sadness or Depression? • How Not to Stress Out in One Easy Lesson
• Living with Loss • Happiness, Optimism, and Longevity • Winter Sunrise • Yielding

5: Our Fears 74

Fear of Aging • Alone, Alive, and Worried • Fear of Being a Burden • Fear of Pain
• Fear of Losing Control • Oh No, Not Public Transportation! • Fear of Dying •

Fear of Abuse • Fear of Being a Bag Lady • Fear of Asking for Help • Fear of the Future

6: Our Love Lives and Relationships 93
Get Hugged! • Expressing Your Sexual Self • When Husbands Die • Long Married • When the One You Love Is Ill • Divorce after 50 • Trusting Yourself in Relationship • Dating after 50 • Choosing Commitment after 50

7: Our Spiritual Self 114
Spirituality and Health • Spirit in the Silence • Obituaries and Inspiration • Journaling the Days • Intuition and Wisdom • Finding Peace • Choosing to Be Authentic • Are You a Goddess? • Liberation from Material Things

8: Our Creative Self 132
It's Never Too Late to Create! • Claiming the Creative Self • Creativity and Health • Dancing from a Wheelchair • Put It on Paper! • Creativity and Longevity • Write a Poem • Write a Book?

9: Our Health 145
Consider the Source • Yoga and Yogurt • Food Is My Friend • The Longevity Test • Why Should I Exercise!? • Where Are My Glasses!? • What You Don't "No" Can Hurt You • What Did You Say? • Uteruses and Vaginas • Sleeping • Physical Disability • Heart Health • Healing Pets • Don't Fall Down! • Coffee and the Pee-Pee Dance • Chew on This • Breasts • Medical Directives

Part III

10: Our Living Spaces 177
Thoughts on Aunt Grace • Staying in Your Home • Gardening and Growing • Color Your World (Feng Shui) • Soulful Living Space • Simplifying • Paint and Wallpaper • Selling Your House • Retirement Living Spaces • Downsizing: Preparing a Move to a Smaller, More Manageable Home • Living Alone and Liking It • Empty Nests with Silver Linings • Clutter: You Can't Take It with You! • Leaving Home

11: Our Families 201
An Easy-to-Visit Elder • Moving to the Circumference • New Grandma • Grandmothering 101 • Distance Grandparenting • Caregiving Grandchildren • Caregiving Our Parents • Parenting "Old" Children • Changing Places: Moving in with Your Kids • Robotic Romeo • Unfinished Family Business • Creating a Family History

12: Our Friends 224
What Matters • The Company of Other Women • Companions on the Journey • Making New Friends and Cleaning Out the Old • When Friends Die • Where Is Everybody? • Class Reunions • The Yeah-Yeah Sisterhood

13: Our Play 238

    Are We Having Fun Yet? • Laughing Out Loud • A Sense of Humor • Challenges
    and Possibilities • Wonder Years • Traveling Adventures • Juicy Curiosity • Our
    Inner Child Never Grows Old

14: Our Work 251

    Reactivate Your Dream • Doing What You Love • Do You Have a Calling? • The
    Entrepreneurial Spirit • Working Retirement • Too Young to Retire • Too Old to
    Get a Job? • What Now?

15: Our Finances 267

    Getting Advice • Giving to Your Kids While You're Still Alive • Helping Your Aging
    Parents • Living Well on Less • Money and Stuff • Planning Retirement • Wealth
    and Happiness

Part IV

16: Looking Forward 283

    Future Dreams • The Freedom to Change • Feeling New Again • Doors and
    Windows • Becoming Human • Harvesting the Past • Get on with Living •
    Starting Over • A Support for the Young • Living Forever • Leaving a Legacy • For
    Future Generations

Study Guide 309
Bibliography 321

Acknowledgements

First and foremost, a big thank you to my talented poet-friend-sister-editor Marilyn Houston for her contributions to this book; to Debra Meryl Cerbini, a brilliant, funny, multitalented assistant-friend and author in her own right who helped make this book a reality; to my husband, Stephen Goldstein, for his support, patience, and love even when I was cranky; to my writers group, Westchester Women Writers, whose feedback on the manuscript was invaluable; to my good friend Tita Buxton for reading the manuscript and sharing her wisdom; to my "Plum Island Ya-Ya Sisters" for helping me keep my sanity and for their encouragement and input; to Nancy and Finlay Schaef, Toni and Skip Lundborg, and the Buxtons for providing quiet, beautiful spaces in which to write; and to my children, Rachel, Aimee, and Ian for being my cheering section.

Introduction

"I have always longed to be old, and that is because all my life I have had such great exemplars of old age, such marvelous models to contemplate."

—May Sarton, *At Seventy: A Journal*

I remember my grandmother and her steadfastness. A pioneer in a new world, she was tough and had to be. A young Swedish immigrant who came to the United States in the early 1900s, she was widowed at 35, the mother of a five-year-old daughter. As I faced some of my own challenges (a couple of divorces, a husband who died, raising children on my own) I could draw some strength from her story. As she aged, I watched her seek ways to grow intellectually (she loved U.S. history, listening to books on tape when she could no longer see well enough to read) and socially (in her seventies she had a boyfriend who was in his sixties!). She walked everywhere and dressed with class. She enjoyed politics, creative pursuits, saving money to buy quality items, teaching and playing with her grandchildren. She died at 101. In Grandma, I had a solid, healthy vision of aging.

As of this writing, I am 56. My sister, Marilyn, who is five years older, also has been an exemplar for me. She's given me glimpses into what I might expect as I age. As mentor and pathfinder for me, she's been an efficient snowplow, clearing and sanding the road ahead of me for safe travel. As grateful as I am to her, the five-year glimpse she offered didn't feel like quite enough. I wanted to know more. What's waiting for me 10, 20, 30, 40, 50 years from now—so I can plan, aspire to greater things, feel some measure of control, and feel a part of an evolving community of women. May Sarton called them "great exemplars of old age" and had them all her life. I realized after entering the second half of my life that other than Grandma and Marilyn, I lacked "marvelous models to contemplate." This book was born out of a search for more role models.

I asked myself questions like, "What will old age and its unknown future with its specter of diminishments of all kinds demand of me? Where is the dignity to be found in it? What can I expect at various stages? What is it now? What will death be? Who and what are we?" Questions with no immediate answers.

Even as our population ages, we are living longer and better lives than ever before. As there is no turning back the clock, the goal as I see it is how best can we live these "golden years," maintaining our quality of life and independence for as long as possible.

We women over 50 are the new pioneers. Colette Dowling in *Red Hot Mamas* says, "Because no previous generation of midlife women had the luxury of seeing decades of productive time roll out before them, we who came of age with the women's movement are in the position, once again, of having to do it for the first time."

According to a *New York Times* article a few years ago, the strong likelihood that baby boomers will reach 100-plus years of age is becoming a reality. Medical advances coupled with technological research are going to extend our life expectancies so much that many of us will easily reach 120. We might become the first generation of women to live 60 or so years beyond menopause! The length of time humans spend in adulthood has more than doubled since the early part of the twentieth century, making it possible for women to have 50 more years with their mates (or without them), 50 more years of watching their children grow old, of career choices, leisure time, physical challenges, opportunities to learn, and 50 more years of trying to fund it all.

In an MSNBC article posted on the Internet entitled "Aging in America," writer Julie Winokur tells us, "The 20th century has given us the gift of longevity. In the past hundred years, life expectancy has increased by three decades, a phenomenon that is reshaping our families, attitudes, work lives and institutions. The proportion of older people in the United States also is growing—by mid-century old people will outnumber young people for the first time in history."

Reaching age 100 is still considered news. However, in the next 50 years, as science, medicine, and bioengineering extend the span of human life, one-hundredth birthdays will lose their mystique. According to the U.S. Census Bureau, by about 2050, the number of centenarians in the U.S. could number close to 850,000 (from just 63,000 in 1900). Then again, if large numbers of baby boomers reach midlife and beyond in good health, that number could explode to something like *4 million* by 2050.

The Next Fifty Years

Gay Gaer Luce writes in an *UTNE Reader* article (November/December 2000), entitled "The Graying of America," that we live in a paradoxical time, that "in the past, respect for the wisdom of the elders was a central tenet of human societies . . . whose elders served as keepers of the cultures' knowledge. But today, in technological countries such as ours, respect has faded into bare tolerance, as we demand that older people act, look, and talk young." Luce says that as America grows old, "this view is bound to change radically. Aging as we have known it will no longer automatically be seen as a time of disability, mental decline, and diminished energy." She posits that many of us will remain alert and active into a second century.

Our families and social institutions will be boggled by a social revolution. I don't want to overload you with more statistics but listen to this: About every seven seconds, a baby boomer turns 50. Retirement is becoming passé, just another word for career change, 80-year-olds are dating, and 90-year-olds are getting college degrees. Thanks to the miracles of medical science, we are experiencing an extension of the human life span. People age 100 or older are surprisingly healthy. We are beginning to see more and more educated, healthy people in our society.

Before the nineteenth century, most people didn't age, they died. Just 100 years ago, few reached age 65. Now there are about 35 million Americans who are 65 and older. By 2030, more than 70 million Americans will be over the age of 65. The number of people over 65 has grown tenfold since 1900.

Esther "Tess" Canja, AARP president, remarked in a June 2000 article in AARP's magazine that "we will be living longer—much, much longer—than we ever dreamed possible. . . . This new era of aging will create an altogether new set of challenges. . . . Already the fastest growing segment of our population is the 85-and-over age group. [The Census Bureau projects that the 85-and-over population will exceed 13 million by 2040.] The next fastest growing group is the centenarians. And now the scientists, with their gene therapies and longevity studies, are predicting a life span beyond the age of 125."

Aging continues to be redefined, and we need new words to define it. In writing this book, I've struggled to find a single word for age 50-plus women that isn't negative. Authorities on aging describe us as being "young" until we're 40, "middle-aged" between 40 and 80, and "old" from 80 to 120. But those terms are broad, and we need better ones that embody the spirit of the woman over 50. Some suggest using the crone archetype, but when I mention it, many women bristle at the word. "Sounds too much like being a withered witch," one woman said.

I find the term "wise woman" appealing. Helen Hayes, first lady of the American theater who died in 1993 at the age of 93, thought we should be called "maturians." For her the word implied there was "still a bit of fight in us." Marilyn, my 60-plus wise sister, doesn't like the words "old" or "older"; I like the word "elder." Some Native Americans use the term "Grandmother Moon," the elderwoman of the tribe. Perhaps we could settle on the term "elderwoman." Instead of the clinical designation of "postmenopausal," we might use the term "opal" coined by Frances Lear, publisher of *Lear's Magazine*. Opals are "Older People with an Active Lifestyle." I like the idea of being opalescent—a gem emitting fire! I also like the idea of changing the word "aging" to "evolving," or as my 78-year-old friend Alma says, "I'm ripening!" I haven't pinned down one word that fits perfectly yet, and I'm still exploring possibilities.

If the world turns in your favor, you could potentially live out all the hidden aspects of your personality, explore your yearnings to see the world or change the world, express your unused talents, serve others, continue your search for love and knowledge—lots of possibilities lie in wait.

I had my grandmother and Marilyn to look to, yet I wanted more. I searched for other stories, experiences, and advice written by women that could inform and inspire me as I entered the next 50 years of my life. I found that the majority of books written for women on aging contained quotes and literary images from the writings of men. However, a woman's experience of aging is different from a man's. Therefore, in the pages that follow you will find heartfelt excerpts, quotes, stories, fun ideas, and serious philosophies *written by women*—women authors and poets and wonderful folks of all kinds who will enrich and inform your aging experience. I hope the results of my personal search will enhance the lives of many of you entering the years of midlife and "beyond"—that you will be inspired in your eldering and your evolving.

Many of the ideas in this book came from 50-plus friends, casual acquaintances, and the women I see as psychotherapy and spiritual counseling clients. The members of the Midlife and Beyond women's group I run and my small personal "Ya-Ya Group" that I take weekends with out of town were inspirational, as were the creative women in the writer's group I founded in 1999. In preparing this book, I spoke with older women from all walks of life: professionals, homemakers, retirees, grandmothers, widows, single women. Most of the issues I write about are common to all of us. The women I interviewed said a book like this is needed.

The Next Fifty Years

Through these women I've come to realize that my aging experiences are not as unique as I had imagined.

We are pioneers of a new age and we are the foremothers of millions of women. For the sake of our daughters and generations of women still unborn, we have an assignment to make clear our role in society: to inscribe the *possibilities of age* on the guideposts to the future. What we create in our mature lives will be our gift to them. Join me in blazing a trail, in creating a legacy of wisdom and strength that can be passed on to the next generation of pioneer women in a new world.

How to Use This Book

The Next Fifty Years contains more than 150 short essays on a broad range of topics that relate specifically to women and aging. Some deal with serious issues, others are meant to be entertaining and lighthearted. You may laugh, you may cry, but most importantly you will realize that you are not alone. I have worked diligently through interviews and research to identify issues that are of particular interest and importance to women as they age.

Each essay is followed by questions with space to write in your reactions, feelings, and/or what actions you might need to take. Studies suggest that writing exercises such as these, which focus on deep thoughts and feelings about life events, can even reduce arthritic symptoms and increase immune function in healthy people. Writing out thoughts and feelings also significantly improves the health of those with chronic illness.

Depending on where you are in your personal journey, the short essay topics may or may not be relevant to you. Some of the worksheets may be difficult to do as you are encouraged to look at issues often ignored. The topic may apply to you today or may apply to you in the future. Read the ones that relate to you at this time in your life and skip the ones that do not apply to you now. For instance, you may not be a grandmother (or a mother) so you would skip the essays on that topic. You are encouraged to respond honestly. Allow time for reflection on each topic and give yourself time to thoughtfully answer the questions.

This book is designed to take you through a process of understanding yourself in relation to aging. I present the more hopeful, exciting, and interesting aspects of aging alongside the more difficult ones. I encourage you to reinvent and re-vision yourself.

The first part provides an overview of the wide spectrum of beliefs held by women and imposed by society regarding the aging process. The second part deals with the inner life of self-image, mind, emotion, fear, spirit, and creativity. Part 3 guides the reader through examining love and relationships with friends and family, how we live, work and play, and manage our finances. Part 4 explores ways to take the experiences and lessons of our first 50 years and use them to plan for the next 50.

The Next Fifty Years is intended to be used as a personal journal, for your eyes only. However, think of it also as a written legacy that, when completed, can be handed down to your daughters or to any younger woman with whom you have a relationship. As you work through and write your thoughts on the pages that follow, you will gain creative, practical ideas for your future. You will gain deeper insight into how you might, with personal integrity, structure your next 50 years.

Part I

1

Thoughts, Cultural Attitudes, and Myths about Women Aging

"In spite of illness, in spite even of the archenemy, sorrow, one can remain alive long past the usual date of disintegration if one is unafraid of change, insatiable in intellectual curiosity, interested in big things, and happy in small ways."

—Edith Wharton, *A Backward Glance*

The attitude that surrounds us is that old age in its most problematic sense starts at 50 or 60. Why is this? I think it's because we still buy into some outdated rule that midlife is the beginning of our decline. This fallacy is based on the equally outdated life expectancy of 47 years or so, which was an average life span at the beginning of the twentieth century. As we all know, the average life expectancy has increased drastically since then, but our cultural attitudes have not.

The one thing we have control over is our attitude toward aging. I have no doubt that the degenerative aspects of the aging process can be substantially retarded by a combination of factors that include attitude, opportunities for service, continuing intellectual stimulation, and good health habits.

Our thoughts directly impact our quality of life. A Yale University professor found that people who think positively about aging tend to live almost eight years longer than those who think negatively. In fact, thinking positively is a more significant life-extender than low blood pressure, low cholesterol, exercising regularly, or not smoking. An article in the *Journal of Gerontology* reported that feistiness makes aging easier, that personal determination to stay independent can help overcome physical frailty. Another study found that an optimistic attitude has a measurable effect on preventing heart disease, for instance.

Living and aging are one and the same. I find it interesting that many people who embrace living still hold on to negative impressions or myths about aging. Living does not stop at a certain year in one's life followed by the process of aging. The sooner we realize this, the sooner we can explore our longevity. To this end (or should I say this beginning?) some of the issues explored in this section deal with accepting change, grieving the loss of youth and celebrating your birthday, cultivating gratitude, enjoying solitude, and embracing a changing tempo of life. The women pioneers of this new age are confronted with common, hurtful myths about aging—that sexuality shrivels up, menopause is a calamity, and intelligence stagnates. This section explores some myths and offers inspiring descriptions of older age and its various stages as written about by women.

When They Were Our Age

". . . we're suffering from an image of aging that comes from a different time. An image that was never anything but propaganda."

—Barbara Sher, *It's Only Too Late if You Don't Start Now*

You can bet on one thing: We won't be doing midlife and the aging process the way our mothers and grandmothers did. Once again we are defining our times. We can be fit, fabulous, and over 50. Although some of the physical changes of midlife and beyond occur at around the same time, for many of us our perception (and experience) of age has changed. Just about nothing in our lives is what it would have been in the lives of women our age even 20 years ago. For the most part, women now are healthier, they expect to live longer, and they are reevaluating their priorities.

We live in a wondrous age. Studies show that most people who reach age 100 do so in surprisingly robust health. Genes may be responsible for about 30 percent of the physiological changes that occur in advanced age, but according to researchers at Harvard University Medical School, the majority of changes are the result of environment, diet, exercise, utilization of available medical care, and mental outlook. With science providing miracle cures for once-fatal conditions, experts on aging even believe that the human life span will someday be increased to 150 years or more.

I love what actress Susan Sarandon said in a *More* magazine article: "It's thrilling to know that around the world, women everywhere are working,

The Next Fifty Years

thinking, daring, creating, making change. I don't know if our mothers ever felt this way about their counterparts—but I have the feeling our daughters will."

My grandmother and my mother were my models of aging women. It was inconceivable to me that I would ever be as old as they seemed to be. Now 56, I realize that I'm the same age as my grandmother was back then, but it feels very different for me than I think it was for her.

In the space below, paste a photo of your mother, grandmother, or other older woman at age 50-plus.

In the space below, tell her how your experience of aging will be different from hers:

_____

_____

_____

_____

_____

_____

_____

_____

Myths to Not Live By

"Of all the self-fulfilling prophecies in our culture, the assumption that aging means decline and poor health is probably the deadliest."

—Marilyn Ferguson, philosopher and writer

Myth: Old women are depressed and lonely.

Truth: We may get depressed and lonely from time to time, but the research shows that the least lonely and depressed women are over 75.

Myth: You become less of a woman as you age.

Truth: Some of the best and brightest women, though past the half-century mark in years, are still climbing the ladder of success in the world.

Myth: Old women have more stress in their lives.

Truth: According to psychologists, older people have more stress-free days than younger ones. That's one of the benefits of aging. The older you get, you kind of realize, "Hey, it's not worth getting upset about the small things."

Myth: Growing older is synonymous with the loss of meaning and purpose.

Truth: Research and the elderly themselves are demonstrating that one's later years can be the richest ever in wisdom and spirituality.

Myth: If you are older and reminiscing about the past, or are becoming garrulous about the past, you are exhibiting signs of senility.

Truth: These recollections are natural and appropriate and their purpose is to resolve conflicts of life and to do a life review.

Myth: The older you get, the faster time passes.

Truth: Mathematically, those proverbial endless summers of your childhood were not even one minute longer than last summer. What's different now is how you spend your summer. Simply put, you have more routines now and routines lend uniformity, which makes it very easy to be oblivious to time.

The Next Fifty Years

Myth: Everyone wants to, and should, be willing to hear our wisdom and opinions because we are older.

Truth: Even though we're older and wiser, we don't necessarily know everything or have all the answers.

Myth: We as women need to be protected.

Truth: Once the protector myth is conquered, women are free to become whole and authentic. Whenever we accept a limiting role, we violate our self.

Myth: Creativity is only for the gifted few and our talents dim with age.

Truth: Creativity is not just for geniuses. It is the energy that allows us to think a different thought, express ourselves in unique ways; it enables us to view life as an opportunity for exploration and it knows no age.

How do you feel about these myths? Write your views here:

_____

_____

_____

_____

Name another myth you have heard about women and aging. What is the truth?

_____

_____

_____

_____

Living in the Present

"Mid-life is a kind of Janus point in the living of our days. . . . It is a time to reflect and digest, to learn and unlearn, and choose a course for the days to come."

—Sarah Smith, *Mid-Life: Coming Home*

How often do you find yourself thinking about some event that *might* happen in the future that causes you to feel anxious and uncomfortable? Doesn't that kind of fretting keep you from enjoying what's available to you in the present? Sure, we have to make plans for our financial and healthcare needs and things of that nature. But once the plans are in place, it's important to be mindful of how you torture yourself out of the present and the beauty it brings.

I find myself thinking about how I will be as a very old woman, and some of what I envision worries me. I wonder how I'll manage if I'm infirm or unable to walk or see well. In those moments, I work at bringing myself back to the present, which is all we are assured of anyway. I keep reminding myself that every moment stands alone, a presence in its own right, a singular visitation that doesn't include the future.

Of course we're getting older every day, but we need something else to think about besides long-term-care insurance and worrying about what our kids are doing when we're home alone. In Sue Bender's wonderful book, *Everyday Sacred: A Woman's Journey Home*, she says, "The challenge is to find even ten minutes when the world stops and for that moment, there is nothing else. How can we bring that quality to what time we have—making that limited time sacred?"

Now take a moment—right now. You are reading this book, sitting in a chair, or on a train, or flying in a plane. Are you comfortable? Does the chair feel soft or hard? What do you see around the room? Are you in a beautiful location? On a beach or a porch? Pay close attention to the small, the beautiful, the meaningful—live in the present—for today, for ten minutes, for an hour. It feels good, doesn't it?

How do you feel about this?

_____

_____

_____

_____

What have you been overlooking in the present because you've been too worried about the future?

_____

_____

_____

Changing Tempo

"I'm . . . trying to do too much . . . I used to be able, as most women are, to do four or five things at once. Do the juggling act. Now, if I can keep one plate in the air, that's good."

—Ursula K. Le Guin, in *On Women Turning 60* by Cathleen Rountree

Seventy-nine-year-old Anne wonders why she's tired. As an alcohol abuse counselor, she sees four or five clients a day, attends training lectures (at some of them she is a presenter), she keeps her own home, and has a wide circle of friends. She's tired because she hasn't learned the fine of art of pacing herself, of dancing to a slower (no-less productive) tempo.

Each week you have 168 hours, 10,080 minutes to work and play. More than likely you spend the better part of your time trying to get too much done—rushing, dashing, scurrying. In the mid-twentieth century, futurists predicted that computers and other labor-saving devices would free up time and transform America into the most leisurely society in history. Exactly the opposite happened.

In this age of rapidly expanding technology and consumerism, how can one fashion a simple, slower paced life? If you buzz from one chore to the

Thoughts, Cultural Attitudes, and Myths about Women Aging

next, from one activity to the next, how can you enjoy your world? For instance, I don't concern myself with slow traffic or traffic jams. I see an opportunity each time to see the world a little more clearly. This is my private time to enjoy the quietness of just being, of stopping to look and to feel and to think, and to indulge myself in a changing tempo.

The rule that we must be accomplishing something all the time is broadcast so efficiently and so early that we internalize it. We struggle with a seditious inner voice that says, "You're wasting time. Get up and do something with your life." Life is going so fast all around us. We're expected (or maybe we expect ourselves) to respond to it in the same way we did when were 20. Does age oblige one to keep up with the latest in technological advances in the culture, such as Internet shopping or online services, in order not to be out of step? Or does one have the privilege by virtue of age of opting out or being selective in one's adoption of this new way of existing? Personally, I prefer pen and paper for personal letters, and meandering slowly through a gift shop, touching and smelling, and smiling at the cashier.

Mary C. Morrison, author of *Let Evening Come,* believes as children leave home, friends move away, and companions die, that we have an opportunity to move into a "discovery-filled solitude" and that we can discover there what our own tempo of living is. Now that my children are out in the world, I'm experiencing this tempo change in my own life. I must admit, I like the new pace.

How do you feel about changing tempo?

_____

_____

_____

_____

Being Vulnerable

"Pay attention to your gut feelings—the gut doesn't lie. And, by all means, don't be afraid to say 'no'!"

—Marilyn Houston, writer and poet

Each year, thousands of Americans over 50 fall prey to a wide variety of house repair, telemarketing, and investment scams. Older women are considered easy targets for con artists because we don't want to be considered rude—we were taught to be nice at all costs. We often lack the skills to end the call when we feel pressure from the person on the other end of the line.

So are you sometimes reluctant to hang up or say, "No, thank you," because you're afraid of offending someone? Many women are at a disadvantage because they live alone or are desperate for money to meet some need. The most common type of frauds committed against older Americans are e-mail, telemarketing, and mailbox scams (which market illegal sweepstakes, bogus charities, unlicensed "health insurers," investment scams, and deceptive lotteries).

Home employment scams are one of the oldest, with envelope stuffing at the head of the list. You're typically asked to write checks for one or two rounds of supplies followed by additional requests to pay for instructions and "advanced" materials. You can kiss goodbye to all you've paid out. Not all business and investment seminars are scams, but many are. One of the key warning signs is being told you'll get rich quickly, that you'll earn up to $100,000 a year, that no experience or training is necessary, that the program will deliver security for years to come, or that it worked for hundreds of others, including the seminar leaders.

Con artists have latched on to healthcare as an easy way to make a buck. Unlicensed "health insurers" promise lofty benefits, with premiums as much as 50 percent below prevailing rates. If you fall for this scam you'll discover that your premiums have disappeared and you're left holding a lot of unpaid medical bills.

These scams are so rampant that the Federal Trade Commission is working hard to prevent us from becoming victims of these schemes. But no commission is a substitute for our own good sense and willingness to say no. Never give money to any business seminar or earn-at-home program until you check out the group with your Better Business Bureau; then get the refund policy in writing and call several previous participants. Local agencies have stepped up their efforts to combat the problem, and several states have laws that make scams against senior citizens a serious offense.

If you think you've been a victim of a scam call the state consumer protection office, the state attorney general's office, the Better Business Bureau, and the police, right away. Don't hesitate because you feel foolish—better to feel a little foolish than a lot sorry.

What will you do if you sense that an offer of any kind isn't on the up-and-up?

_____

_____

_____

_____

Aging Can Be Fun?

"It really IS funny to see an adult looking all around the room for her glasses without noticing that they are on top of her head."

—Helen Heightsman Gordon, *Age Is a Laughing Matter*

Is it possible that growing older can be fun? Perhaps our negative expectations have something to do with our experiences. Since my friend Joan turned 40 (12 years ago now), she laments the aging process every chance she gets. She defines it solely as the breakdown of the body and its functions. As a result, she seems to be creating more discomfort for herself all the time— more aches, more pains, more visits to the doctor. She has been for years expecting life to be miserable when she came closer to 50. Joan reminds me that "F-U-N" are the first three letters of "funeral"!

On the other hand, my over-70 friend Tita talks of what is exciting, fulfilling, and fun in her life. If she has aches (and I'm sure she does), she doesn't focus on them. She travels, she reads, she laughs, and she nurtures her relationships with her friends, children, and grandchildren.

As for me, I'm looking forward to becoming more outrageous, aches and

The Next Fifty Years

pains and all. In *Be an Outrageous Older Woman*, Ruth Harriet Jacobs says, "As I grew older, I learned that if you are outrageous enough, good things happen. You stop being invisible and become validated." Right on, Ruth!

If I someday need to walk with a cane, it won't be an ordinary one. I'll paint it red and white to look like a candy cane. If I must use a walker it will be equipped with a bicycle horn. Beep, beep—out of my way! If the arthritis in my hands bothers me, I'll wear green polka-dotted mittens indoors in the winter. Aging can be an outrageously validating experience if we stop focusing on the funeral and focus on the fun instead.

What expectations do you have of aging?

_____

_____

_____

_____

Describe something outrageous you could do to make aging more fun.

_____

_____

_____

_____

Accepting Change

> *"Life is change. It will change around you if you don't change with it."*
>
> —Helen Gurley Brown at age 78, *The Late Show*

Everything is in a constant state of change—our bodies, homes, families, spiritual connections, the world around us. Sure, we can use our energies to fight and resist. But there is something bold and strong about surrender. Change is inevitable, and resisting it causes our souls great sorrow and pain. While we're so busy resisting we risk missing out on the potential for enormous joy. There probably isn't a day these days that you're not acutely aware of change. Your body is changing, your family and friends are changing, your strength and speed of mental processing are changing, and your priorities are changing. How are you dealing with these changes? Denial? Acceptance?

As for me, if acceptance means "approval," I say no, I don't approve of some of what happens as we age. If acceptance means I will work change into my life, then I say yes. If change means painful loss and disappointment, I say no, I don't want any of that! (And do I have a choice?) If change means growth, forward movement, and a refreshed attitude, I say yes. If acceptance means I will let myself go as I age then I say no. Frances Weaver, author of *The Girls with the Grandmother Faces,* tells us it's our attitude toward all these changes that's most important. "The sincere desire to lead a productive, interesting life at any age depends upon our own imagination and acceptance of new ideas."

Tell yourself that if you embrace this time of dynamic change you will feel more peaceful. That you're on an adventure. Say yes to feeling peaceful—and say yes to adventure.

How do you feel about this?

_____

_____

_____

_____

How is your life changing?

_____

_____

_____

_____

Age Grief

"You know what surprises me most as I cycle through the five stages of age grief? How did I, a bona fide child of the 60s, end up sounding like my parents?"

—J. Eva Nagel

Shock, denial, anger, bargaining, acceptance—these are the identified stages of grief. When it comes to age grief, I find I am reluctant to believe the grief associated with aging is similar in its stages to the grief one feels when someone is dying. Yet after considering this a while, I believe it is.

One day I woke up to find that my youth, reckless or not, had become middle age, that I was clearly and inevitably moving toward old age. Now, that's a shock. Denial set in as I tried to stay up as late as I used to and when I tried to work all day in the garden without a rest. Certainly I had always been able to push myself when it came to physical work, but now I had to devote shorter blocks of time to the same activities. I didn't stay in denial long because I was too busy being angry. Angry that it was different now. Angry that my back and legs hurt after stooping over the weed patch. Angry that I was now falling asleep during Letterman!

Bargaining? Not sure about that one. I still haven't tried to bargain with the higher power to make me young again or fit. No, I haven't said, "God, if you give me the energy and looks of a 30-year-old, I'll pledge more money to charity." I may do this at a later date. For now I'm working on acceptance. You see, I had planned on aging naturally, with grace and faith, with a nonattachment of sorts. I knew reincarnation and heaven were possibilities so I wasn't so concerned with death. I don't take myself too seriously. My eyes are focused and wide open. And still some days I miss aspects of my younger years.

We will all mourn our youth to some degree. What is hopeful is that if we identify where we are in the process, then allow ourselves to move through it, we will come out the other side energized and ready to face the future.

How do you feel about this?

_____

_____

If you feel you're grieving for your lost youth, what stage of age grief are you experiencing? What can you do to move through it?

_____

_____

_____

_____

Ages and Stages

"For me, there's something so liberating about this stage of life. It's not that you know more, necessarily; it's that you accept not knowing and experience a different kind of ease."

—Susan Sarandon, *More* magazine, February 2002

People are staying healthy and living longer and the old stages of life no longer hold. According to some scientists, a woman who reaches age 52 today and remains free of cancer can expect to live to age 92. In *New Passages*, best-selling author Gail Sheehy tells us, "People now have three adult lives to plan for; a provisional adulthood from 18 to 30; a first adulthood from about 30 to the mid-40s and a second adulthood from about 45 into the 80s." She says that the key to mastering this passage is to do something people generally haven't done before, which is to plan for this second adulthood.

It is heartening to know that other women have philosophical thoughts about aging. There's a broad range of expectation, capability, and emotional experience in aging—what is true for one person may not be true for another. The voices of the women quoted below will give you an idea of the diversity of experiences. The quotes represent some of my favorites from a variety of authors on the various ages and stages of a woman's life.

50-60 Years Old

"Old folks today are doing more than anyone ever thought they could. Why, when we were children, folks were knocking on death's door after turning fifty. Sixty was ancient . . ."

—Sarah L. Delany, *On My Own at 107*

60-70 Years Old

"Sixty years bring with them the privilege of discernment and vision: a capacity to behold, in the blink of an eye, the sweeping panorama of a life fully lived."

—Cathleen Rountree, *On Women Turning 60: Embracing the Age of Fulfillment*

70-80 Years Old

". . . when I think that I'm seventy-eight, I think— how could that be? I just don't feel like whatever I would have thought seventy-eight would feel like. I just feel like myself."

—Betty Friedan, *Life So Far*

80-90 Years Old

"I am more and more aware of how important the framework is, what holds life together in a workable whole as one enters real old age, as I am doing. A body without bones would be an impossible mess, so a day without a steady routine would be disruptive and chaotic."

—May Sarton, *At Eighty-Two: A Journal*

90-100-plus Years Old

"I must tell you at once that I have become over ninety in the course of writing this book, and yes, being over ninety is different. . . . I can say with all honesty, I'd rather be a very old woman than a very young one."

—Rebecca Latimer, *You're Not Old until You're Ninety*

"Somewhere along the line I made up my mind I'm going to live, Bessie. I guess I probably don't have that much longer on this Earth, but I may as well make the best of it."

—Sarah L. Delany, *On My Own at 107*

How do you feel about these quotes?

_____

_____

_____

_____

Which quote do you relate to the most and why?

_____

_____

_____

_____

Write your own quote here:

_____

_____

Aging Is Another Country

"Actually, aging, after fifty, is an exciting new period; it is another country."

—Gloria Steinem

Never before in human history have we had the possibility of living beyond 100 years. To be truthful, there are days when that prospect excites me. Is it possible that I may have so much more time to realize a few of my dreams, finish reading all the books I bought, make new friends, have new adventures, repair screwed-up relationships, and organize (once and for all) my front hall closet?

Then there are the days when the thought of 100 (or even 90) gives me the willies. All that sagging skin, all those dead friends, all those lost umbrellas and gloves, pills to take, young know-it-all doctors to undress for, and insurance forms to fill out.

I'm in a constant debate with myself: should I age into decrepitude or call the cosmic taxi for a fast ride to the Other Side while I still have gray matter that functions, and while I still look and feel pretty good?

Horace B. Deets, AARP executive director, tells us that it's time we "learn how to deal with the longevity bonus productively—The new reality of aging is that we must all plan and prepare to live long, healthy and productive lives." So perhaps we should keep our hearts and minds open to ways we can debunk the myths, fight the worn-out stereotypes—become warriors of a kind. I think about being a warrior and I want to take a nap. Then I shift to a burning curiosity that asks the question—what will that "other country" have in store for me? And for heaven's sake, what will my passport picture look like?

How do you feel about this?

What would you like to accomplish if you live to be 100?

_____

_____

_____

_____

An Attitude of Gratitude

"It is in our later years that we are often able to give our most meaningful consideration to values, to refocusing our priorities, shifting our outlook and developing a sense of gratitude for the richness of life."

—Connie Goldman and Richard Mahler, *Secrets of Becoming a Late Bloomer*

Self-help gurus have lectured to us about gratitude for years now. How much more harping are we willing to endure before we take their advice to heart? They're right, you know. Gratitude for even the smallest of things can magically shift a tough day from gray to sunny bright just like that.

Here is a case in point. I wake up mopey, eyes crusty, hair sticking up at right angles, the result of a crummy night's sleep (postmenopausal night sweats, husband snoring, cat jumping on my feet). Groaning, I slide out of bed. Then, barefooted and stiff, I slog across the icy kitchen floor, reach for the coffeepot, realizing as I lift it that I'd forgotten to set it up the night before. Now I must endure the noisy coffee bean grinder, put the coffee into the filter, pour water up to the line. I am waiting for what feels like three weeks for the damn java to trickle too slowly. I so desperately need my sanity, my caffeine. There is no joy in my life at this moment.

I remember the self-help gurus and decide to "do gratitude" while I wait. I decide to focus on the positive, like Ruth Turk who wrote *The Second Flowering*: "To my amazement, I continue to find each decade of my lifetime more rewarding and exciting than the preceding ones." So let's see—I'm grateful I have a husband (snoring and all). I'm grateful I have a house and warm bed to sleep in. I'm grateful for my sticky kitchen floor, and I'm grateful the floor is cold because it reminds me that I've forgotten my slippers (which I'm

The Next Fifty Years

very grateful I have). I'm grateful for my coffeemaker and the aroma of fresh beans. I'm thankful for the nose that enables me to smell the coffee brewing.

Got the idea? You can spend the day grousing because you forgot why you walked into the living room or you can be grateful for the legs that got you there.

How do you feel about this?

_____

_____

_____

_____

What are you grateful for today?

_____

_____

_____

_____

An Attitude of Solitude

"There have been times . . . when I have longed for solitude, and it took some hard lessons for me to learn that I needed to be what I had thought was selfish; that I need to take time to myself to write, to go to the brook, to be."

—Madeleine L'Engle, *The Irrational Season*

I remember my 89-year-old grandmother sitting in a chair, doing nothing. Her face looked tranquil. She didn't look depressed. When I asked if she was okay, she said she was reliving a wonderful, fulfilling time in her younger years. At that time Grandma still led a busy life—seeing friends, going to her club, reading books, caring for her grandchildren. Yet she knew how to be still. She was comfortable with solitude.

I was once afraid of solitude, afraid of my internal sounds. I found our extroverted society encouraging me to constantly communicate in some way. I've come to realize that my need to pull away from other people is as universal as the urge to connect. As I age, I find I need time to be in touch with me. Pagers, cell phones, e-mail, and fax machines give us the ability to be in constant touch with each other. I have a need to know myself, to sort things out, to regroup. I want to understand how I think and feel and where I want to go with my life.

Time alone will serve to restore your integrity, allow you to think about your beliefs and what you value most. A self-imposed quiet can fertilize your creative side as ideas emerge, long buried by the daily rush. Alone time replenishes energy so when you resume interacting with others, you do so with renewed insight and strength.

Don't wait until you have a whole day or week free to incorporate a bit of solitude and reflection into your day. Try simple pleasures—walk in the park, sit in a room and listen to music, sink into a warm bath, meditate for ten minutes, pet your cat. If you aren't used to being alone, you might feel a little bored at first. Stay with it. After a few minutes you may like it.

How do you feel about this?

_____

_____

_____

_____

How can you create more solitude in your life?

_____

_____

_____

_____

Birthdays

*"I want to tell people I'm 75 instead of 65
so they'll think I look great for my age!"*

—Patti Dudyshun, astrology counselor

Just before my fiftieth birthday I suffered a concussion and damage to my neck in a car accident and consequently missed having the celebratory party I had envisioned. When I finally started to feel well enough to give a party (it took two years) I decided I would celebrate my fiftieth at age 52. Now when my birthday rolls around, I feel each birthday is once again my fiftieth because, having survived that accident, I'm so glad to be alive.

At my fiftieth birthday party (which I celebrated at 52) I bought party hats and noisemakers for my guests, and bubbles to blow. I plan to celebrate my fiftieth over and over until I'm 100. I will never deny my true age, but when I send out the invitations to my birthday party each year they will say, "I am celebrating my fiftieth again," because that was the year I realized how precious and precarious life is.

Gifts are another issue. Don't we have enough stuff at this point!? My over-70 friend Alma told me we should all "get a hobby so your friends and your kids will know what to buy you. Then you won't end up with a bunch of extraneous nonsense." My friend Clarice told me, "When I turned 50 I asked my husband to give me a gift that was older than me and he gave me a bonsai tree!"

Negative feelings abound on the issue of birthdays. Author Mary McConnell said in *Still Dancing* that "turning sixty sneaks up on you, like a difficult guest you know is coming . . . and suddenly sixty knocks at the door." Some women I've spoken to barely enjoy their birthdays anymore. That's a shame, because for most, birthdays were so special when they were younger. Other women dread celebrating their birthdays because they don't like calling attention to their age.

Not everyone is negative when it comes to celebrating their years. On her sixtieth birthday my friend Patty told me, "I love celebrating my birthday. The attention is on just me—all day! I've got no problem saying how old I am. I was born on July 25th so I've always celebrated the entire month—starting with July 4th. On reaching 60, I'm feeling a new freedom—total permission to be me. If I want to do anything, good or bad, the decision is totally mine. I

Thoughts, Cultural Attitudes, and Myths about Women Aging

feel just fine saying 'no' if I don't want to do something. In recent years I've rented a house on the beach where I celebrate my birthday with my friends. My time at the beach house gives me a sense of peace and calm and brings me back to who I am."

Try not to think about the accumulation of your birthdays. It's how you feel that matters. Consider spending your birthday in a way that feels best to you—with others or alone. Or try one of these:

• Do something daring like rent a convertible and drive with the top down, or arrange for a hot air balloon ride.

• Throw yourself a party for an in-between birthday—like 57 instead of 60.

• Before your birthday, buy a beautiful journal. Fill every page with positive memories, and things you're proud of, then give it to yourself as a birthday present.

• Spend part of the day meditating and reflecting on your life.

How do you feel about this?

_____

_____

_____

_____

What would you like to do for your birthday this year?

_____

_____

_____

_____

Saying What I Mean

"Perhaps one can at last in middle age,
if not sooner, be completely oneself.
And what a liberation that would be!"

—Anne Morrow Lindbergh, *Gift from the Sea*

As Gloria Steinem said, "Women may be the one group that grows more radical with age." Lynne Zielinski tells us in *Chocolate for a Woman's Spirit* that "like autumn fruit, I've mellowed and thrown off inhibition to say what I mean." So has my sister, Marilyn Houston, who wrote this poem:

Cookie Cutters

Aaaah, the scene opens . . .
whether you like it or not
rain punctuates puddles marking cadence
for a spotty spring ballet of fools
it's a goose-step two-step,
so very tiring especially if you do it right

I'm a sun-dancer with a tie-dye mind
running from clones in Cadillacs
drones in cathedrals, perpetually
harping we've fallen from grace
they're expecting the worst
and it never disappoints . . .
so many blank faces, so little time
how can anyone deny God's sense of humor
while under the sublime influence of Heaven
or is it advertising?
I declare war on snobbish university poets
their self-proclaimed perfectionism incensed
that we don't follow their rules,
their pentameters, particulars and perpendiculars
ha, you can't stop me now with your parameters,
there's a lot more where that came from
and I'm not about to do it your way
even if your power trip
IS bigger than I am
'cause I gotta voice

Thoughts, Cultural Attitudes, and Myths about Women Aging

Listening to your inner voice makes it possible to start living more authentically—to speak with your own true voice and from your own system of values and beliefs. Telling it like it is invites women to go beyond the superficial injunctions of the culture—to be pleasant individuals, to be invisible or nice. As we age it becomes even more important to assert our power in relationships and work. It's time to become more direct and more outspoken.

As writer Maxine Myers once said, "I no longer consider silence a virtue. Speaking up is OK, and speaking up louder is even better in some cases."

How do you feel about this?

_____

_____

_____

_____

If you could broadcast a belief about a political, personal, or world issue that you haven't had the courage to express, what would it be? (You might want to write it out as a poem or a speech on a separate piece of paper.)

_____

_____

_____

_____

The Decision

"I want to make a terribly important point. People decide to get old. I've seen them do it. It's as if they've said, 'Right, that's it, now I'm going to get old.' Then they become old. Why they do this, I don't know."

—Doris Lessing

Perhaps you've entered a time in your life when your strength or abilities have diminished. You were active in one pursuit or another your entire life, and now you're not as able (or completely unable) to continue those activities. It's probably time to find a new purpose, a new reason for living, and it's time to find new opportunities that will cause you to stretch and grow.

Where do you begin? Begin with a decision. As Doris Lessing tells us, we *decide* to get old. That means we've got some control over this passage into the next 50 years.

As for me, about four years ago I decided that I'm not aging—I'm evolving. Don't you just love the sound of that word? Evolving, revolving, involving, solving, and resolving not to "get old." You can evolve until you die (and maybe even beyond that, but that's another book).

I have an idea. Decide to be old one day a year when you go for your physical and the doctor says, "You know, at your age . . . you should, etc. . . ." The other 364 days a year when you're not in your doctor's office, put your energy into evolving. Here's another idea. Gather up all your health statistics (cholesterol numbers, etc.) and put them in a file. You know the statistics I'm talking about—those numbers that remind you you're aging. Then visit your statistics once a year or so (unless your health really depends on another regimen). Remember, you have a choice—you can make the decision to put meaning and excitement into your life or you can decide to be old.

How do you feel about this?

_____

_____

_____

_____

What unhelpful decisions have you made about being old?

_____

_____

_____

_____

Waiting

As I age I feel I am at the same time getting better at waiting and more impatient with it. When I barrel through my days at high speed, I'm increasingly aware that I miss the nuances of the moments that are only available when you are still.

I remember my grandmother. No matter what the occasion or who was coming to take her out, she was always ready to go an hour ahead of time. She would sit patiently by the front door, coat on, purse held tightly on her lap, waiting. I used to feel uncomfortable seeing her sit there so long, but it has occurred to me lately that it was an activity for her. That perhaps she used those quiet, unhurried moments as an opportunity to meditate, be in the moment, to experience more fully what was happening inside and around her.

I am feeling that I want more "slow time" these days, more patience, more internal peace while I wait. When I was younger, waiting was an anxious, trying to make time move faster activity. I wanted "fast time." I couldn't *wait* for Christmas, my birthday, to turn 12, to turn 21. I couldn't *wait* until graduation, until my baby was born, until the tulips came up, until summer arrived. I couldn't *wait* to get married, to buy a house, to receive the blouse I ordered, to see my boyfriend on Saturday night.

When I can manifest "slow time," I know I'm living in the present moment. It becomes a balancing act between learning how to wait and not passively waiting for life to show up. Peaceful waiting means trusting that I am in the right place and that all is evolving in the universe as it was intended. So I will learn to wait, not for life to pass me by—but so that I can see life's unfolding more clearly.

How do you feel about this?

_____

_____

_____

_____

The Next Fifty Years

Part II

2

Our Self-Image

"Most important, I will learn that being old is a badge of honor, not a reason to hide in shame. I will refuse to be invisible!"

—Finy Hansen, *New Age Magazine*, Nov/Dec 2001

For many women, self-image and self-esteem begin to decline with age. They feel invisible. They feel young on the inside but not in their outward appearance. They find it takes more effort to maintain their looks and their bodies.

With so much emphasis placed on appearance by our society, the scariest part of aging for many women is that they now have to rely on *who* they are rather than on what they *look like*. They, like me, will have to ask: Now that my youth is behind me, who am I? I had to ask myself: Am I so attached to my younger looks that I've misplaced who I really am at 56? I felt estranged from my body, and the weight gain I experienced after menopause was weighing me down.

As far back as I can remember, I've been able to eat what I liked without gaining too much weight. I'd burn it off running errands and chasing children. Imagine my amazement when this metabolic miracle ended just as I was on the cusp of 50. Though I had not changed my eating habits one iota, suddenly I was gaining, and gaining until I discovered I was 40 pounds overweight. I tried on everything in my closet and donated anything without a stretchy waistband. I didn't even try on the jackets I knew I wouldn't be able to button.

At one point I told myself I wanted to be like Ruth Harriet Jacobs, author of *Be an Outrageous Older Woman*. Ruth likes to wear outrageous clothes. She writes, "I am a woman of size but refuse to hide in black or navy blue. I wear bright colors and wild styles rather than apologizing for age or taking up sizable space in the world."

Where do I fit now? Some of the older women in my neighborhood have white hair, some are arthritic and stooped, some look like they've given up. Sometimes we smile at each other. But I wonder if they consider me one of their own? Or have I fooled them with my dyed hair, my expensive cosmetics, and my gym clothes? Sometimes I feel like an impostor, and part of me wants to deny kinship with these older women. I want to be in the club, but I want to look good, feel good, project health.

Should we totally ignore the image we project? Of course not, but as older women, we are also much more. There are two authors that I particularly admire for their insight and wisdom concerning women's self-image. In *Journey to the Heart,* Melody Beattie says, "Love how you look, smell and feel. Love the color of your eyes, the color of your hair, and the radiance of your heart. Love how you laugh. Love how you cry. Love your mistakes, and love all the good you've done."

Elizabeth Cady Stanton said, "Be kind, noble, generous, well-mannered, be true to yourselves and your friends, and the soft lines of these tender graces and noble virtues will reveal themselves in the face . . . in a personal atmosphere of goodness and greatness that none can mistake. . . . We cannot be one thing and look another. . . . There are indelible marks in every face showing the real life within."

This section will help you explore the key issues of redefining your older self-image, and what questions we need to ask ourselves about what constitutes a healthy self-image.

Becoming Invisible

"Many women approaching 50 don't feel glamorous; they feel invisible. . . . I think they mean sexually invisible, but if they send out the right vibes, they won't be."

—Judith Krantz

Judith Krantz brings up a good point. What kind of vibes are you sending out? I remember the first time I heard the "invisibility" indictment. I was sitting with a client who was 15 years older than me at the time (which made her about 56, the age I am now). She had just gone through the healing process from a difficult divorce and was ready to start dating for the first time in 30 years. She felt invisible and unnoticed at social events even when she was dressed well and coiffed to the nines. I recall thinking to myself that I would never feel that way.

Yet these days, I've come to feel the invisibility I was so sure I would never experience. I thought it would be more upsetting than it is. I thought my self-esteem would plummet and that I wouldn't feel sexy or desirable anymore. It's actually quite a relief for me because so much of the pressure to be fabulous in all ways has lessened. Mary McConnell in *Still Dancing: Life Choices and Challenges for Women* reminds us that "growing older is not a reason to develop low self-esteem. Many women find new confidence and self-assurance after fifty."

That's what I've decided is worth working on—a new confidence and self-assurance. I've joined a gym and Weight Watchers and have lost a few pounds. I've also had my "colors done" and a makeup consultation that is helping me to feel better about how I look. Am I still invisible? Probably, maybe. But I'm not invisible to me. I matter, and I am clearly here, on solid ground, feeling confident and in tune with my body. You will undoubtedly develop extremely low self-esteem if you have relied on your looks to give you a sense of value. If you think that's the only way you are seen, then be prepared to become invisible and stay that way. I love what Marianne Williamson says in *A Woman's Worth:* "As we age, gorgeous young hunks may or may not be interested in us any more. For that matter, men our own age and older might not be interested anymore. My response to that is 'so what?'"

Here's a goal worth setting—say to yourself: "I will arrive at the point where I am comfortable with who I am and as invisible as I choose to be."

How do you feel about this?

_____

_____

_____

_____

What can you do today to feel more visible to yourself?

_____

_____

You Don't Look Like a Grandma!

"There are more grandmothers alive today than at any other time in the history of the world. However, today's grandmothers don't look like grandmothers."

—Lois Wyse, *Funny, You Don't Look Like a Grandmother*

What is a grandmother supposed to look like? Mine looked sweet and had small, strong, arthritic hands. Her skin was transparent and loose crepe paper skin decorated her outstretched arms. Her eyes twinkled like Mrs. Santa Claus and when she got mad her face reddened, her high-pitched voice poised to cut you in half. After the scolding she would give you a big hug, then, wrapped in a handmade apron, she'd produce stacks of thin, buttery Swedish pancakes. She cooked *everything* in butter, yet she didn't weigh more than three bags of groceries. Did she look like a grandma? You bet. More than that, she acted like one.

Grandma was the one you could go to with the stuff you didn't want to share with your mother. She wasn't as judgmental. She played cards with us, and Parcheesi and Chinese checkers. She taught me how to sew with a thimble and knit scarves.

I have five grandchildren. Do I look like a grandmother? I would like to think not—yet, what am I so worried about? I sure would like to be more of a grandmother, not as concerned about every little wrinkle, ache, and pain, but more concerned with being the one the kids come to with their problems. I'd like to worry less about my postmenopausal weight and be more available to play gin rummy or Nintendo. I'd like to be less concerned with how much my skin is sagging and focus more on giving the best hugs in the world.

If you're lucky enough to be a grandmother, ask yourself, "Am I more preoccupied with looking and staying young than I am with being a caring and generous grandmother?"

How do you feel about this?

_____

_____

_____

_____

What can you do to be less focused on your appearance and more engaged with your grandchildren (or other family members)?

_____

_____

_____

_____

Who Is That Old Woman?

"Sometimes I look in the mirror expecting to see the body, the face of my youth because I remember her. She's still in me."

—Melody Beattie, *Journey to the Heart*

Sometime after turning 55 I remember waking up one morning to the birds singing outside my window and the smell of coffee brewing. I believed it was going to be a perfect day until I struggled to my feet, hand on my back, and hobbled past the full-length mirror on the bedroom door. "Who is that old woman? Am I still in there?" I wondered.

Then I remembered something else that made my day. In doing the research for this book I had read that after 50, our tissues start drying out. This is one reason weight actually drops after 55. Of all things, they tell us that around 65 our noses and earlobes elongate. Oh my. Floppy earlobes and long noses. However, our biological clocks tick at wildly different rates and no two women will age in exactly the same way. So, while some of you are drying out and losing weight at age 55, others of you may not experience nose droop until you're 80.

Not wanting to deal with all this information on my own, I called my friend Deb for some consolation. She listened while I moaned and groaned about my inevitable decline with age. She jokingly replied, "Let's just kill ourselves and be done with it!" That's one way to end your concern and I don't recommend it. I think it's important to have a more upbeat approach. I'm considering this: when my ears are longer, my dangle earrings will swing better, and if my nose gets longer, at least it will be drier and I won't have to stoop as far to smell the flowers.

How do you feel about this?

_____

_____

_____

_____

Write down some positive, encouraging statements about how you are aging:

_____

_____

_____

_____

Sagging Faces and Liver Spots

"An 82-year-old friend of mine decided to buy herself some nips and tucks. Her daughter said that at her age it would just be rearranging the deck chairs on the Titanic."

—Peg Bracken, *On Getting Old for the First Time*

The fact that plastic surgery and skin care technology have made it possible to turn back the hands of time in a very visible way continues to feed our insecurities. These days you can erase a decade from your looks if you choose to. The question is: How do you choose to live peacefully with your looks when the pressure to do just the opposite is so overwhelming?

Liver spots have nothing to do with your liver. Those flat, brownish spots are the result of years of sun exposure. They're bigger than freckles and appear on the faces, hands, and arms of fair-skinned people. That's me! The medical name for them is solar lentigo, but they're also called senile lentigo, not because you're getting senile but because the name comes from the Latin word for "old." Oh lordy, lordy—senile liver spots.

My 62-year-old friend Mary told me, "I'm in great physical shape for my age. But a lot of people were telling me how tired I looked. I had a face-lift and had those bags removed from under my eyes. So now my face looks as young as my body feels. Believe me, I'd do it again without hesitation." Thanks to cosmetic surgery others don't have to see us as middle-aged or older. With special contact lenses, you'll never give away your age by needing your reading glasses to cut your steak. A little hair coloring from the box can "wash that gray right out of your hair" and advances in plastic surgery make it possible to erase years from your face and body. But as Lois Wyse reminds us in *Funny, You Don't Look Like a Grandmother,* "As for cosmetic surgery, until they figure out a way to make a woman's hands look as young as her face—who's she kidding?"

Are we too obsessed with staying young? A middle-aged Japanese woman I spoke with said she thinks American women are more afraid of getting old than Japanese women are. Evidently, in Japan plastic surgery is popular with young women; however, they use it to enhance their looks, not to remedy the effects of aging.

We clearly make ourselves miserable. At a certain point in our lives we find ourselves engaged in fighting back against every ounce of weight gain or every hint of a wrinkle. We engage in so many efforts to hold back the ravages of time, until finally at some point we give up and forget about the whole thing. That's when we become happy again. Even sagging faces look beautiful when adorned with a smile. And liver spots? Oh heck, call them freckles if it makes you feel better.

How do you feel about this?

_____

_____

_____

_____

High Maintenance

". . . if women can learn to surrender the seductiveness of youth and to value themselves by other than adolescent standards of beauty, they can explore the dignity of 'elder beauty' and reclaim the right to age without stigma."

—Z. Schachter-Shalomi and R. S. Miller, *From Age-ing to Sage-ing*

Despite my usual optimistic outlook, I've collided with age and its required upkeep. I wish I could report that I arrived at these high-maintenance years with complete grace and dignity, but that's not true. In the last decade or so, baby boomers have surreptitiously redefined aging. If I want to I can dress like a teenager, inject collagen into my wrinkles, color away the gray hairs, replace my old dry nails with acrylics, and liposuction the belly rolls. But thinking about all of this makes me just plain tired!

Do you find yourself examining your skin for possible melanomas? They look like brown or black crusty growths that show up from nowhere as you age. It's a good idea to have your skin checked by a dermatologist once in a while. But try not to obsess about every little bump. What about that cellulite? I don't think any amount of maintenance can cure that. Just don't look in the three-way mirror in the dressing room anymore. Remember, as you age, everyone around you is aging too. This should make your particular maintenance issues seem less daunting.

Have you noticed that the heroines of your favorite movies are discreetly, yet beautifully, older women and that they just keep looking better? Well, consider that it's part of their job to maintain themselves and that they've got thousands of dollars of income to spend on themselves. So go easy on yourself and try to enjoy a maintenance-free day once in a while.

How do you feel about this?

_____

_____

_____

_____

What particular maintenance activity are you obsessing about that you could let go of?

_____

_____

_____

_____

Feeling Young Inside

"'It's hard to admit to being old, isn't it? I keep thinking, How'd this happen? Sixty-one! When I was young I looked at people this age and thought they must feel different inside. . . . I thought they would just naturally feel like they were wrinkled up and bent and way far along.'
"'It don't feel that way, though, does it?'
"'No,' Alice says . . . 'It feels regular.'"

—Barbara Kingsolver, *Pigs in Heaven*

Lately, there isn't an older woman I meet who doesn't say, "I feel much younger than I look." When I see photographs of myself, or videotapes of TV programs I've appeared on, I can't relate to the image I see. I feel so much younger inside than the images reveal. I'm not aging on the inside. I think we've all had that experience at one time or another. May Sarton wrote in her journal *At Seventy* that "seventy must seem extremely old to my young friends, but I actually feel much younger than I did . . . six years ago."

A devotional book I once read talked about being aware of what "young" really is—"young" is "eager, curious, dauntless, willing to explore, to struggle, to be foolish as the world goes, caring, trusting, open and brave." Being an older woman is all of those things as well.

Regardless of what the outside looks like, inner beauty is a beacon, like a beam of light that reveals something undeniable about a woman's core. That beam brightens her entire self, introducing a definition of beauty broader than anything that preceded it. So what is this light? More than any other quality, I believe it's the ability to experience pleasure that makes a woman desirable and beautiful. Pleasure in her work, in her friends, in the food she eats, maybe even pleasure in her stressful days. Isn't it a woman's unconscious pleasure in herself and her pleasure in others that allow her to lean forward and let go, and make the rest of us want to lean in toward her, wanting to connect?

If beauty comes from the core, then what part do looks play? Should we just nurture and support our inner selves and forget about the outer? Are the two, as we sometimes fear, mutually exclusive? Will we forever be guiltily battling the exterior with the interior, presuming that one is bad, the other good, and forgetting that both are integrally linked? They are linked. We make a mistake if we see inner beauty and outer beauty as somehow antithetical, demanding that inner loveliness stand on its own without even moisturizer or a bit of blush. Self-nurturance doesn't negate self-worth but rather bolsters it.

The older woman with inner beauty knows this and she is resolute. She has made tough choices to become who she is. I think we appear much more beautiful and youthful to others if we can say, "Here I am, with all my flaws, passions, vices." Show me inner beauty and I'll show you a woman who has rid herself of the superfluous, both inside and out, who has kept what she needs, refused the rest, and regretted nothing. This culling, often called centering, is at the heart of every system of spiritual enlightenment I know of, and the result is what finally accounts for inner beauty's insistent glow. Several coats of black mascara won't interfere with your spiritual life; I promise. Even the most evolved among us still has to face the day.

How do you feel about this?

_____

_____

_____

_____

The Next Fifty Years

Old Bodies, New Again

"I never thought I'd live this long. No one in my family did. I eat well. I keep away from fats. And you've got to exercise."

—Constance Poirier, 102 years old, *New Age Magazine*, January/February 2000

Even if you have never exercised or eaten right, you can start now. I don't want to be one more nagging expert telling you to exercise and get in shape. Let me just tell you my story instead. At 54 years old and 5 feet 9 inches, I weighed in at a hefty 236 pounds. Too much Cozy Shack pudding, Raisinets, and Rice Krispie Treats and a lot of sitting around on my duff. I joined Weight Watchers and the gym and lost 30 pounds. I never thought this old body could feel new again.

I read in an issue of *Bottom Line Personal* that our muscles have "memory." According to Avery Faigenbaum, professor of exercise physiology at the University of Massachusetts, if you exercise regularly and then stop—even for years—your muscles will respond more quickly when you start exercising again than the muscles of someone who never exercised. Even if you stopped working out years ago, your body will help you get back into the healthful habit.

When it comes to taking control of your physical self, I like what actress Helen Hayes once said: "If you look at all the assembled data on the decline of the human body, you'll come to the inevitable conclusion that you are, if not in command, certainly in charge of supervising *how* you age."

It's important to get out and do something and to remember that even an old body can feel new again. It doesn't matter how long you've had negative thoughts about your body, you can begin to make a change today.

How do you feel about this?

_____

_____

_____

_____

Proud of Our Wrinkles

"Growing older is a nice feeling. It's something people don't talk about. They only talk about wrinkles."

—Isabella Rossellini, actress

So you want to laser away wrinkles, lift those droopy eyelids, tighten that turkey gobbler neck, or suction fat from your middle? Many women are fearful of looking older (mainly because they feel younger) and are willing to put up with the pain and expense to look like they feel. In this country, cosmetic surgery has increased by 75 percent in recent years.

You can share your retirement money with a plastic surgeon and get a few tucks around your eyes or chin or both. Or invest in some expensive magic cream they proclaim will erase your wrinkles. Not me. I'm kind of proud of my wrinkles—wrinkles that reflect the years of my youth, that say I've struggled hard to be a good mother, an aunt, a grandmother; that I've taken pride in my home, my garden, my ability to keep ten plates in the air; that I've worked hard to become a writer, a gardener, a baker of bread, a singer, and a therapist. My wrinkles are the stripes that represent my years of service. Each one represents a laugh, a sorrow, a ray of sunshine, or concern for another that etched character and strength into my soul. Plus, they get me a seat on the bus and a discount at the movies.

Our facial lines show that we've lived. I admire the character and intelligence of faces that are no longer youthful. The intelligence of a mature face can be much more compelling than the insipid beauty of someone whose main asset is a tight face with no crow's feet.

I find myself studying the slightly crinkly eyes of my older friends as I try to develop some appreciation for my own fine lines. I've taught myself, through meditation and therapy, to treat my particularities as gifts. I also refuse to compare myself with other women of any age. Instead of trying to look young, I'm aiming for looking unique.

Millions of women are aging and refuse to show it. Botox and collagen injections, laser treatments, chemical peels, and dermabrasion are all attempts to erase the real beauty and intelligence of the aging face. Not for me! I'm not planning on erasing anything.

Remember, your wrinkles aren't visible invitations to an old folk's home. Older, grayer women than you are spending their face-lift money on going back to school, taking yoga classes, and taking trips to Australia to watch the sunrise.

How do you feel about your wrinkles?

_____

_____

_____

_____

Looking Good

"Even when you know you'll be completely alone for a day or more, put on your makeup, comb your hair, and dress in something comfortable, but nice-looking. It's what that does for you, not for others. It makes you feel good."

—Judge Judy Sheindlin ("Judge Judy")

My friend Sari Martin, a professional personal image coach, says, "No matter what your age, plan an event every day for which you need to get dressed—a trip to the grocery store or post office, a walk with a grandchild, or tea with a friend. Many women get lazy, especially after they retire, and end up wearing their bathrobe for half the day, or slipping on a pair of sweatpants and a loose T-shirt. Loose-fitting clothing affects your posture and the way you walk. It negatively impacts your energy. Making the effort to get dressed says you feel good about yourself."

She also says, "If it's your quest to look younger—avoid 'super-young' looks. *Seventeen* magazine isn't your resource guide. Avoid too tight or too short. Avoid shoe heels that are too high. Avoid too bare when it comes to skin-revealing outfits. Check the style and length of your hair. A new hairdo can shave ten years off your birth date."

I think the key to looking good and feeling good as you grow older is to keep trying new things—new hairstyles, wardrobe colors, exercises, even new foods. Do some experimenting and enjoy the results. See a professional about your makeup. Ask for advice on a makeover. Try different stores. See if the various cosmetic wizards agree on what your best colors are. Many offer free makeup applications. Try different looks and see which suits you best.

Listen, do not worry too much about your age. Learn to dress with flair. Take a style class and learn which colors you should wear to brighten your complexion and which ones leave you looking washed-out. How about a new perfume? Try two or three different fragrances. Switching scents will make you feel fresh and different.

A facial massage will make your face look more relaxed. For heaven's sake, get a pedicure. A pedicure, complete with a foot and leg massage, relaxes you and makes you feel special right down to your toes.

If you're interested in looking gorgeous, consult an older woman. My friend Patti D. says, "The greatest invention since control-top pantyhose is the pink lightbulb."

We are bombarded with images of perfection. Our culture celebrates youth. Women now feel they can't afford to look mature. There's pressure to have plastic surgery. If you look rested after a vacation, friends ask, "Who did your eyes?" In Europe, the educational system tells young people to study now so they can have fun later. Being an adult is something to aspire to. In America, it's the opposite. Adulthood is when you stop being attractive, stop having sex, and start being responsible. No wonder people delay growing up. They think it will be the end of enjoyment. U.S. film actresses in their fifties have trouble finding good parts, while European actresses look their age, yet remain symbols of elegance and attractiveness. I think a thickening body attains more stature, and bone structure becomes more interesting when it is no longer concealed by the pudginess of youth.

It seems some of our celebrities have the right idea. Consider actress Isabella Rossellini, who said, "I don't do anything to look younger; this is one battle that you will lose eventually. It is more becoming to accept the unique characteristics that come with age. Women who stay true to themselves are always more interesting and beautiful." World-famous model Iman said in an interview that "after a certain age, thinness is not attractive. You'd be surprised, but five extra pounds can make you look healthier, younger, more attractive." Laura Mercier, renowned makeup artist, says, "Age is sexy because it brings wisdom and knowledge of yourself. As for style, you know what looks good on you. You've learned from your past mistakes; you are not distracted by trends."

Let's face it—you look good when are comfortable with who you are—that's what shows and that what makes you beautiful.

How do you feel about this?

_____

_____

_____

_____

Now Who Am I?

"I love being old . . . because I am more myself than I have ever been."

—May Sarton

As my grandmother aged, her life became less about what she looked like and more about who she was becoming. As I enter more fully the second half of my life, the journey is bringing with it a different dimension of growth from the first half. The insurance tables tell me there are more years left in which to get to know myself better.

If you're trying hard to stay young, you're stalling out your own self-discovery, pretending you're still in life's first half. You may have decided that your entry into life's second half will begin at a later date, like when you reach a certain age. Or perhaps you have accepted that you're in life's second half, but still struggle with the unanswered question, "Now who am I?"

In trying to answer that question, you may be so terrified that you attempt to make superficial changes to your old persona while avoiding any profound change or self-understanding. You may change the old mask cosmetically, buy new clothes, or change your hairstyle. But nothing can hide your changing self. You can't *sort of* begin this quest. Either you do, or you don't—and if you're beyond 50, the time to decide has arrived. If you do not dare to grow, the ghost of the first half of your life will haunt you.

Suzanne, a 52-year-old artist and writer, told me, "I'm not going to apologize for my age. I'm going to wear my hair long and gray if I want to just because it feels good. I intend to feel my feelings and think my thoughts. I will be who I am."

Perhaps you've had the experience of suddenly realizing that the structure of your life does not seem to fit you and you don't know why. Relationships you chose may now seem unfulfilling. Your aging face suddenly seems prominent. Material things that once brought pleasure may now seem totally inadequate. A lifestyle that once seemed satisfying or tolerable now grates on your nerves. Goals that were clear may become overwhelming or blurred.

For some women, their identity was wrapped up solely in their love relationships. Have you lost yourself in a long-term relationship or marriage? Is your self-esteem dependent on how your mate feels about you? If you spent half your life focusing on him so much so that you don't know what your own wants, needs, and desires are, it's now time to commit to knowing who you are. In accommodating themselves to others and focusing on relationships, many women neglect building a sense of themselves as distinct and valuable individuals. At midlife, a woman's most obvious sense of herself may be in terms of her relationships with others as daughter, wife, mother, or employee. When she realizes this, the question of who she is *apart from* these relationships often becomes difficult to answer.

You may be 50 and already deeply engaged in the quest; or you may be 80 and still resisting it. This is because your chronological age is based on clock time; the quest moves through soul time, which many people encounter for the first time only in the second half. Soul time has less to do with calendars than with the deepest dimensions of life.

Ruth Raymond Thone makes this declaration in her book, *Women and Aging: Celebrating Ourselves:* "As an aging woman, I must give myself permission to be who I am, even if that is not culturally approved or productive. I need time to be tired, quiet, sick, sad, old, and unproductive. I want to affirm who I am at each moment of my life, not wishing for another time, another self, nor molding myself to fit an inner shape that no longer serves."

Helen Nearing, age 89, author, champion of human rights and the joys of simple living for over 60 years, gives this advice in *Wise Words for the Good Life:* "Live. Adapt to other people. Breathe in and breathe out in an aware fashion. Be aware of where you are, what you are doing, and why you are doing it. Live day to day. That's what we're here for, to find our way through the fog."

If it feels uncomfortable to ask yourself the question of who you are now that you're older, honor your resistance and follow the signs leading to intensity. Your enemy is shallowness. If it feels safe, it's probably not the right path. If it scares you, it probably is. In this second half of your life, you have another chance, another opportunity to learn who you are. I think it's important to

The Next Fifty Years

accept yourself unconditionally. When you do, you'll be surprised at how comfortable you become no matter where you are in your life.

How would you define yourself now?

_____

_____

_____

_____

_____

_____

_____

_____

_____

_____

_____

Strong in a Youth-Obsessed World

Atomic Mother

I'm here now to tell it like it is,
in spite of your arrogance, your ignorance.
Love and determination keep me strong
in a youth-obsessed world that doubts my value.
I refuse your chronic misperceptions, definitions
that try to keep me small and powerless.
Classic Mother, that's not all I am, I promise you.
Simple acts of love revealed my power
even before I held the universe in my womb.
I've given all to those I love, so don't assume
my gender renders me diminished.
At any given hour, I'd kill or give my life for them,
the ones I love—without hesitation.

I've got a strength that goes beyond your understanding.
Should I not be seen as Goddess in your eyes?
Is my power to create too much for you to bear?
Am I less than clever for the wrinkles on my face?
Am I less than the shadow of your perfection?
Take a look at your own reflection
. . . and your lies.

—Marilyn Houston

We women of the 1960s and 1970s were forerunners and barrier breakers. As a group, we Renaissance women (both working women and stay-at-home wives/mothers) were joined by others who felt exhausted and vacuous. We had courage in the face of resentment, we stood up to be shunned and satirized. We were some of the first women to rescue ourselves instead of waiting for the Knight on the White Horse (or in the White House). We are strong.

How to do you feel about Marilyn Houston's poem "Atomic Mother"?

_____

_____

_____

_____

What can you do to feel stronger and more confident about your self-image and about the person you have become?

_____

_____

_____

_____

3

Our Minds

". . . our sweetest life, our truest life, is with us always—beyond the senses, ever rooted in consciousness."

—Marsha Sinetar, *Don't Call Me Old—I'm Just Awakening!*

As the nation's baby boomers age, the number of Americans with late-life mental or emotional issues is expected to climb. Millions of women over 50 already struggle with the changes, losses, and stresses of growing older, and their numbers are increasing sharply as the nation's population ages.

Put simply, I don't want to lose my mind—or my way home for that matter. It reassures me to know that some mental challenges such as depression, chronic anxiety, and dementia are not part of normal aging. However, most of our mental and emotional challenges are manageable. The good news is that we've had a revolution in our understanding of the brain and we now know that the brain is constantly rebuilding itself throughout life. More good news—the past decade has seen the emergence of a full-fledged specialty in medicine called geriatric psychiatry. This practice is aimed specifically at the diagnosis and treatment of mental and emotional problems that affect older people.

Leading researchers in neuroscience and in psychology are continuing to discover more about the nature of consciousness, memory, emotions, creativity, dreams, and other mental phenomena, as well as how and why the brain ages. Their answers suggest that some of these mysteries may be largely solved within our lifetimes.

This section contains essays with suggestions on how to keep the brain active by pursuing continued learning and exercises to help increase memory. With a somewhat humorous twist, we will take a look at misplacing things, loss of memory, those annoying senior moments, the mind/body connection, and the effect that menopause, with its hormone depletion, has on the brain.

Your Brain Is a Muscle

"Women who believe in themselves are enhanced by the sum of their years. We are repositories of the experience and wisdom of our time."

—Betty Nickerson, *Old and Smart: Women and Aging*

A once-common notion that the brain declines with age is completely false. Scientists have demonstrated that new brain cells can actually be generated in adults, proving that the brain continues to grow and actually improves with age. Until very late in life, older people tend to perform better than younger ones in certain areas, such as vocabulary, numerical skills, spatial orientation, and interpersonal problem solving.

The brain is like any other muscle in the body and it must be exercised to stay in shape. Since the brain depends on the cardiovascular system to supply it with oxygen-rich blood, it is crucial to remain physically active as you age. Lack of physical exercise is likely more responsible than age for declining brain function. Although it makes up only 2 percent of your total body weight, the brain consumes roughly 20 percent of the oxygen you breathe.

Another way an unfit brain can be whipped back into shape is with an exercise program for the brain called neurobic exercise that encourages you to try different things and develop new hobbies. Here are some exercises from Lawrence C. Katz, Ph.D., author of *Keep Your Brain Alive*:

• Take a different route to work
• Turn pictures on your desk upside down
• Shop for food at an ethnic market
• Sit in a different seat at the dinner table
• Have a blind wine tasting
• Go camping
[I like the wine-tasting suggestion.]

Take care of your health and your brain will love you for it! Eat a nutritious, balanced diet. Adequate amounts of vitamins B_6, B_{12}, and folic acid are particularly important for memory, as well as the antioxidant vitamins C and E and beta carotene. Have regular checkups because memory problems can be caused by cardiovascular conditions; thyroid dysfunction; depression;

diabetes; lung, liver, or kidney problems; and drug side effects. See your eye doctor, too, because changes in sight or vision can contribute to memory problems.

What steps will you take to exercise and care for your brain?

_____

_____

_____

_____

Senior Moments

"Losing our minds is more frightening to most of us than death."

—Sallirae Henderson, *A Life Complete*

Don't you just hate it when you find yourself standing in the middle of a room saying, "Now what was I on my way to do?" Mary C. Morrison tells us in *Let Evening Come*, "It takes longer to remember things. . . . But if we wait— a name, a place, an event will come to mind, swimming slowly to the surface, like a fish rising." That reminds me of the day I wanted to remember to bring up frozen fish for dinner from the basement freezer. I wrote the word "FISH" on a sticky note and stuck it to the front of my T-shirt. When my assistant showed up later that day, she had a good laugh when she saw the note still stuck to my shirt and no fish defrosting in the kitchen. Talk about fish rising slowly!

It's hard to imagine that memory is composed of a collection of dendrites or neurological connections that make up an organic function subject to injury or atrophy. But that's what's in our heads. So keep in mind (no pun intended) that not all memory lapses are normal. See your doctor if you forget things much more often than you used to—forget how to do things you have often done before—get lost in familiar places—forget where you've been for a few hours—have substantial trouble learning new things—lose awareness of daily events—start to repeat phrases or anecdotes during the same conversation. Simple memory lapses are probably not due to an organic problem, so lighten up on yourself. In our many years on this planet, we've stored a great deal of information in our noggins. Frankly, we need to let go of some in order to make room for more.

So what can you do to minimize senior moments? One study of people 55 and older who consumed one to three alcoholic drinks a day showed they had 42 percent fewer cognitive difficulties. Maybe grandma was right when she sipped on her sherry for "medicinal purposes." But remember, it's not a good idea to start drinking if you don't already.

Most importantly, try to be less judgmental of yourself when a "moment" happens. If you're worried, tell your doctor what's going on (ask her if a little wine might help). In the meantime, decorate yourself with sticky notes in bright colors to match your outfits and accept that you will have a senior moment from time to time.

How do you feel about this?

_____

_____

_____

_____

What will you do to help yourself remember things?

_____

_____

_____

_____

Mind/Body Connection

"My body has been giving me strong hints for some time now that things are changing. The body knows. It's the mind that's so reluctant to accept the phenomenon of aging."

—B. J. Bateman, in *Our Turn, Our Time: Women Truly Coming of Age* by Cynthia Black (ed.)

My 76-year-"young" friend Alma once told me, "Don't say, 'I must be getting older' because your body hears you and then it reacts that way." Alma's right. Scientists have developed new molecular and pharmacological tools that have made it possible to identify the intricate communication network that exists between the immune system and the brain, a network that allows the two systems to signal each other continuously and rapidly. These systems guard against infectious, inflammatory, autoimmune, and associated mood disorders. These systems also "hear" everything we "say."

What we think about pain also has an effect on the amount of pain we're in. I remember reading about a 102-year-old woman who said that she had a pain in her finger and decided it might be arthritis. She said to her finger, "If you're trying to attack me with arthritis, nothing doing!" She massaged it and massaged it, and a couple of months later her arthritis pain was gone.

Someone once asked me a very important question: "How old would you be if you didn't know how old you are?" I'm not sure, but I think I'm around 40. If my body keeps getting messages from my mind such as: "I'm too old to walk that far," "I'm not young anymore," "Women my age don't do that," then I take the risk that my mind is going to "hear" me and my body is going to obey.

Try some mind/body exercises like meditation, yoga, and slow, deep breathing to get centered and in touch with your body. Most importantly, watch what you tell yourself about aging—your body is listening.

How do you feel about this?

_____

_____

_____

_____

Name one body/mind exercise you would like to try:

_____

Make a list of positive messages you will give your mind and body today:

_____

_____

_____

_____

Losing Things

"You can decline to look for items you misplace. Let them find you. It simplifies life enormously to have three of everything like eyeglasses or car keys or canes or umbrellas."

—Peg Bracken, *On Getting Old for the First Time*

Peg Bracken has a point. When it comes to eyeglasses, for instance, it's a good idea to have several pairs. In fact, I need my glasses to find my glasses sometimes. Perhaps the best way to keep from losing things is to not have too many things to lose, but that's another story (see "Liberation from Material Things" in chapter 7).

I don't think losing things is necessarily a result of the weakened cognitive abilities that come with age. We lose things primarily because we don't pay attention to where we're putting them in the first place. When I'm intent on wanting to remember where I've put something, I'll say out loud to myself, "I'm putting the car keys on the dresser." Saying aloud where I've put something seems to create the necessary neural pathway for retrieval later. I don't care if anyone hears me talking to myself. They may think I've gone crazy, but talking to myself is better than going nuts trying to find my stuff.

Another way I help myself keep track of things is to have what some organizers call a "landing spot." My landing spot is on the dining room table. This is where I put anything that has to go with me in the car when I do my errands;

that's where I put mail to go out, my keys, cell phone, purse, bag for the Goodwill bin. One woman I know places everything she wants to remember to take with her directly in front of the door so she can't get out without tripping over her stuff.

Remember, losing things doesn't mean you're getting old and losing your mind. You just need to pay attention, develop a system, put things in the same place each time, and buy three of those items you just can't live without.

How do you feel about this?

_____

_____

_____

_____

What system of keeping track of things would work best for you?

_____

_____

_____

_____

Is It Menopause or Mental Pause?

"During menopause we are literally moving into our wisdom years, where we can access a broader range of knowledge and can synthesize things rationally."

—Christiane Northrup, M.D., *Health Wisdom for Women* newsletter

Like many issues related to women's bodies, until recently menopausal transition, which can take from six to 13 years, has been considered a somewhat less than appropriate topic for everyday conversation. As a result, we've been denied access to our mother's and grandmother's experiences and wisdom. Among the topics connected to menopause that we hesitate to discuss is the feeling that our brains have gone soft.

For some women, the hardest part of the journey is what feels like a lessening of intelligence or mental abilities. Some midlife and older women worry that their intelligence is diminishing because their thinking has become foggy or sluggish. Foggy or fuzzy thinking emerged as a term of reference in the 1990s to describe the sometimes confused thought processes that many women experience at menopause and midlife. It could be attributed to physical changes in the brain, emotional disturbances, stress, and hormonal shifts, among other factors.

Doctors may dismiss memory loss and difficulty concentrating as a result of stress or, in menopausal women, low estrogen levels. Those symptoms can also mean you have hypothyroidism (underactive thyroid) or that you are depressed. Both can be treated effectively, so it's best to have a full physical to check on these things.

Medical textbooks say estrogen appears to function as a mild vasodilator to increase blood flow within the brain. As a woman transitions through menopause, researchers have documented differences in the actions of estrogen on neurotransmitters and receptors in the brain. These changes are most pronounced during the years a woman is moving through the menopause transition.

Some good news: It appears that certain processes and functions of the brain make permanent shifts after menopause so that many women become more creative later in life because the parts of their brains that handle creativity become more active (see chapter 8, "Our Creative Self"). Take life a little slower, create something, and take some action to ease your mind.

How do you feel about this?

_____

_____

_____

_____

What are you willing to do to "ease your mind"?

_____

_____

_____

_____

Memory, What Memory?

"There is one anxiety about aging that I think we could well do without, and that is when we can't remember a name, or can't recall what it is we have started to do. . . . It does not mean we are getting senile . . . we are in a state of overload."

—Eda LeShan, *It's Better to Be over the Hill than Under It*

As you age, you may find your memory is not as good as it used to be. All is not lost, including your memory. There are a number of simple strategies to keep your memory working to capacity and your mind sharp. Aerobic exercises can improve memory 20 percent or more. Use to-do lists and sticky notes, of course. Get enough sleep. Keep your stuff organized or reduce the amount of stuff you've got to keep track of. That should help a lot. And my favorite: talk to yourself as you do a task. Don't worry who's listening. Try it. Talking out loud focuses your attention on what you're doing and will make it easier for you to remember later.

Researchers have made some interesting findings. In a May 2001 *AARP Bulletin*, Vicki Freedman of the Philadelphia Geriatric Center said, "More than 10,000 people age 70 and older in a 1998 study performed better on memory tests than others tested in 1993." The University of Michigan ran the battery of tests and discovered that "the greatest improvements were found among people in their 80s and those who had never graduated from high school."

Our skin begins losing its memory after 40. They say that if you pinch hard the back of your hand it will smooth out in two seconds. By 65 it will take about 20 seconds. Imagine that—as we age, even our skin forgets where its going! But don't stress about that. You need to lower your stress in order to boost your memory because hormones released under stress interfere with the brain's ability to remember detailed information.

Saint-Exupéry said that in our old age we will sit under the sheltering branches of the tree of our memories. I just love that image—now if I could just remember where that tree is.

How do you feel about this?

_____

_____

_____

_____

What steps will you take to bolster your memory?

_____

_____

_____

_____

Continued Learning

"As you get older, you learn to modify your activities and the demands you make on yourself. The trick is to continue to learn, to challenge yourself."

—Helen Hayes, *Helen Hayes*

Perhaps one of the best ways to keep your brain healthy is to take some classes, either at a university or by enrolling in a local continuing education program. Some of you may hesitate going to school because you might feel old enough to be the mother or grandmother of your fellow classmates. I suppose some of those younger students may be at a time in life when they want to get away from their mother. I say, don't worry about them. You are entitled to learn and grow at every stage in your life. In fact, I've heard younger students say how inspired they were by someone older in their classes.

Have you heard about Elderhostel? At this writing it's the world's largest educational travel organization for people age 55 and older. Last year, a quarter of a million people took more than 10,000 Elderhostel programs in 100 countries. Clearly, there's a strong demand for this kind of affordable adventure travel. The instructors are professionals and the accommodations are usually high quality.

The Next Fifty Years

What about getting a degree from home? Take a look at www.lifelong learning.com. You'll find a database of accredited courses there. I think it may be more stimulating to attend a class with other students if you can. The class discussions can be the most interesting part of the learning experience and you may make some new friends in the process.

Perhaps you put off college or pursuing additional training while you raised your children or supported your husband. Now it's your turn. One of our greatest challenges as human beings is to live life without regret. Have you put a dream on hold because you didn't have the skills or education? Take the chance to rethink your future, to listen to that still, small voice within you— the voice that has, from time to time, whispered a dream to your heart.

How do you feel about this?

_____

_____

_____

_____

Do you think going to school is a good idea for you? If so, what would you like to study?

_____

_____

_____

_____

Brain Growth

"If I manage to learn something new, I glow with a pleasure that life seldom gave me in youth, when I took all of this for granted. There is nothing like old age to make one aware of the marvels of the human body and mind."

—Mary C. Morrison, *Let Evening Come: Reflections on Aging*

According to experts, society's knowledge doubles every ten years and the average person today has already absorbed five to ten times the experience of their grandparents. I say knowing five to ten times what my grandparents knew is quite enough, thank you. And I suppose we could just stop there and not learn anything new and be content knowing what we know. But as I age I don't want my brain to stop growing altogether, so I've made a decision to keep it stimulated and challenged.

Master detective Hercule Poirot, the hero of many of Agatha Christie's novels, boasted repeatedly about the power of "the little gray cells" in his head to solve tough mysteries. When I mentioned this to my friend Ellen, she told me that she must be getting more comfortable with age because she's now allowing the color of her hair to match her brain matter.

I'll bet you didn't know that older people score higher than younger people on some mental tests. The theory is that older folks make fewer errors because the age-related decline in memory function makes them "less likely to be led astray by misleading contextual information." I'm not sure how to interpret this. It feels like the researchers are giving with one hand and taking with the other.

Never mind all that research data—try one of these brain-growing activities and enjoy your life more:

- Learn photography or a foreign language.
- Memorize a poem.
- Learn to play an instrument.
- Play new games (Chess and Scrabble are great for the brain).
- Read some great literature.
- Redecorate your environment.
- Try solving crossword puzzles (start with the easy ones).

The Next Fifty Years

How do you feel about this?

_____

_____

_____

_____

What actions will you take to keep your brain growing and active?

_____

_____

_____

_____

4

Our Emotions

"People with positive outlooks, who continue to connect themselves to the future and marshal their energies to defeat creeping depression or entropy, are far more likely to extend their Second Adulthoods into satisfying later lives."

—Gail Sheehy, *New Passages*

By about 50, we've amassed a hoard of wisdom that should carry us through the rest of our lives. But too often, difficult emotions get in the way and accessing our stored wisdom becomes a challenge. We may lose our optimism for life to bouts of situational depression. Losses begin to pile up as we age. We are challenged to keep our emotions stable and, fighting for our lost youth, we forget how to yield gracefully.

In addition to the normal aging process, another factor that influences our emotional lives is our health. The condition of your health (see chapter 9, "Our Health") will of course have an effect on how much you do in your life, how you do it, and how you function emotionally. If you build on and focus on the strengths you *do* have, your emotional life will be less affected and aging will become more satisfying. The emotional aspect of aging is a challenge, but it is also an opportunity for enormous growth.

This section offers a pathway through the emotional "mind-field" of aging. You are encouraged to write responses to essays that deal with emotions that some women face, such as the role of optimism in aging, how to detect depression, deal with changing moods, and the effect of stress in our lives, as well as living with and managing life's inevitable losses.

Bad Moods

"Tears do come occasionally into one's eyes, and they are more often than not a good thing. At least they are salty and, no matter what invisible wound they seep from, they purge and heal."

—M. F. K. Fisher, *Sister Age*

Who hasn't had a bad mood? Moods seem to show up like an ambush, unannounced, uninvited, and unprovoked. Often moods are tied to a particular circumstance, such as if your Social Security check didn't come on the day you expected; your gray roots grew back before you had a chance to buy more hair color; you looked in the mirror to find your cellulite is dropping toward your knees. Things like that can put anyone in a foul mood. Other common sources of bad moods include recent illness, loneliness, boredom, unrealistic expectations, failure to accomplish a goal.

Bad moods certainly magnify the trivial annoyances of life. Like running out of tea bags or coffee filters, forgetting your toast in the toaster, and tripping over the cat while looking for your glasses (the seventh time today). The unprovoked moods are the most annoying, I think. It's much easier when we can blame something or someone for the mood we're in, but it's not always kind or helpful.

Take time to analyze what was happening before the bad mood occurred because this may give you a clue to the remedy. Keep a mood journal where you track your ups an downs for a while. Note the circumstances (where you were, with whom, what you were doing). Try to catch and record the internal events that preceded them—thoughts, memories, fantasies. Then imagine how a nondepressed person might feel in these circumstances, remembering the difference between a feeling (it passes quickly) and a mood (it lasts). You can take this journal to your doctor or to a therapist if you think your bad moods are getting in the way of you enjoying your life.

Or try one of the following to help ease your mood:

• Shift the focus away from your bad mood by doing something for someone else.

• Eat a little bit of chocolate. It prompts the release of serotonin, the brain's natural chemical upper. Eat it slowly, savoring the sweetness and texture. (I prefer walnut fudge.)

- Play with a toy. Two of my favorites are Slinky and Play-Doh. Something as simple as a yo-yo or windup toy can help distract your mind and relax your body.

- Get active. Take a quick walk. Walking prompts the release of endorphins and provides a change of scenery that may distract you from your problems. One of my personal favorites is walking in the woods or near the water with an 89-cent bottle of bubble soap in hand, blowing bubbles as I go.

- Listen to upbeat music—rock, heavy metal, rap, reggae, ragtime (my sister loves the heavy-metal group, Metallica). Sing along to the music; belt it out—it helps.

- Ask a friend to help you cheer up or allow their positive outlook to "infect you." Avoid people who bring you down.

Add some of your own:

_____

_____

_____

_____

Is It Sadness or Depression?

"But what was happiness? Had she been happy? . . . one was happy at one moment, unhappy two minutes later, and neither for any good reason; so what did it mean?"

—V. Sackville West, **All Passion Spent** (Lady Slane, an 88-year-old character)

The World Health Organization came out with something they discovered sometime in the 1990s: that depression, although higher in women, falls dramatically after 65 years of age. Hooray! Another benefit of growing older is that we are growing less depressed.

On the other hand, are you finding that you've lost your usual spark and sense of humor? Have you stopped going out? Are you avoiding your friends? Do you stare dully at the TV? Do even the grandkids fail to cheer you up? You might tell yourself that you're just slowing down, but there could be another reason. A growing number of Americans are dealing with serious depression, a draining condition that can ruin the quality of life and often goes unrecognized in older people. Experts say the problem, if not brought under control, will only worsen as baby boomers age and confront life changes and losses that can cause depression.

Clinical depression is more than sadness, the blues, or a reaction to grief. Depression is a medical problem, like hypertension or diabetes. Furthermore, the condition isn't what I would call a part of normal aging. Still, some 90 percent of depressed older adults don't get relief because they are reluctant to seek help or because their doctors don't recognize their illness. Nine out of ten of us receive no treatment. Truth is, doctors often miss the diagnosis because their depressed older patients usually see them for somatic complaints instead.

Minor depression usually lifts on its own. But you're likely to need active measures to banish a lingering case. As a first step, get adequate sleep, eat a nourishing diet, and spend more time with friends and family. Exercise is also a powerful antidote. In more persistent cases, therapy can reveal the underlying causes of depression and can help reverse negative attitudes and find better ways of handling problems. Antidepressant medication can also help.

Some of the symptoms of a depression that needs treatment are: you feel you are worthless, empty, unloved, hopeless; you no longer enjoy things, feel very tired and lethargic, feel nervous, restless, or irritable; you are unable to concentrate, cry frequently, sleep more or less than usual, have persistent headaches, stomachaches or pain; and in extreme cases, you have thoughts of death, especially suicide.

Generally, psychiatrists believe most depression is biochemical, but many of them don't accept a specific link between hormone deficiency and depression. Women with obvious hormonal issues are often treated with antidepressants. Some are even given shock therapy. Often the underlying hormonal component of their depression is misdiagnosed.

Depression does not reflect a character weakness or a personal failure. Indeed, depression often occurs in older women who have lived a normal and productive life. Some mature women develop depression because of brain changes resulting from medical illnesses or hormonal changes. Loss of a loved one, social isolation, physical pain, and other discomforts may precipitate or exacerbate depression in persons with such brain changes.

Sudden depression in someone over age 50 may signal a "silent stroke." So watch out for that one. Silent strokes don't result in classic symptoms (severe headache, dizziness, loss of motor skills) but are often the precursor to full stroke.

You might also develop depressive symptoms if your thyroid gland (an endocrine gland in your neck) is out of whack, so make sure you ask your doctor to do in-depth blood work. If you are diagnosed with hypothyroidism (underactive thyroid), it can be easily treated.

How do you feel about this?

_____

_____

_____

_____

If you suspect you're depressed, what action will you take to address it?

_____

_____

_____

_____

How Not to Stress Out in One Easy Lesson

"If you have lost your husband, your home, your health, your car, lowered your income due to retirement, and moved away from your established community, you are building your stress points right off the chart."

—Mary McConnell, *Still Dancing: Life Choices and Challenges for Women*

One of the best ways to burn out is to pile one stress on top of another. Of course, we can't avoid stress altogether. However, you probably have more control over the timing of stressful events than you think. For instance, if you've recently lost your husband, don't immediately sell your home. If your health is diminishing, don't panic and run off to an assisted living facility. Think things through. Delay responding if you can. Handle one circumstance at a time. Find support, get feedback, slow down!

If predictable stressors are coming your way, try not to face them all at once. Sandra A. Crowe, author of *Since Strangling Isn't an Option*, suggests you "give yourself a break. Choose a task to postpone or delegate—cancel your dinner plans so you can enjoy a restful evening. Give yourself permission to recharge. Meditate, take a catnap, or just close your eyes and visualize comforting, enjoyable experiences."

Remember, there are enormous benefits to keeping your stress under control as you age. Our bodies are in direct communication with our emotions and stress has an effect on all the major organs. Here are some other ways to control stress:

- Invite a grandchild or neighborhood youngster to a tea party. Being around a child can give you a new perspective.

- Get a massage. A massage can help you feel loved and nurtured. It can also ease the muscle tension and aches that sometimes accompany a bad mood.

- Play with your pet or volunteer at the local pet shelter.

- Most important—create a loving, supportive network of friends. Not having a close friend or confidante is as detrimental to your health as smoking or carrying extra weight.

How do you feel about this?

_____

_____

_____

_____

What can you do to reduce the stress in your life?

_____

_____

_____

_____

Living with Loss

"Until I can mourn the loss of a dream I cannot be comforted enough to have vision for a fresh one."

—Madeleine L'Engle, *The Irrational Season*

As we age, we will all experience two kinds of losses: gradual and sudden. The gradual losses are things such as your eyesight not being what it used to be, or realizing that over time your walking has become a little less stable. Sudden loss may come in the form of a stroke where you are suddenly disabled, or the death of a spouse or friend. Each month, nearly 12 million people mourn the loss of a loved one, and mourners often experience the most desperate times in their lives.

Then there is the inevitable loss of status, sometimes gradual, sometimes sudden, as we age. Changing from wife to divorcee or widow, or from worker to retiree, is a status passage that involves a kind of death of the old self.

As we age it is difficult for some women to accept the gradual loss of a youthful appearance (see chapter 2, "Our Self-Image"). We look in the mirror and see new wrinkles or frown marks—our once familiar face now portrays a road map of our journey through life. One woman I interviewed was grieving the loss of her youthful looks and lamented, "My hippie days are gone. Remember that natural look? It's gone!"

One way to manage loss is to gain strength and meaning from others' stories. For example, find a biography or autobiography or video of an artist, playwright, or author who has experienced loss. You will see that in most cases, the negative energy of loss was turned into a creative pursuit with a positive outcome.

Going after what we have lost is a natural response, but what are we going after? Perhaps we are "going after" the meaning of loss in our lives. As I said in my earlier book, *I Wasn't Ready to Say Goodbye*, "Grief is not something we 'get over' or heal from as if it were an illness. It is a journey to a new stage of life. The goal is not forgetting or resolving. It is reconciling yourself to that loss and discovering some kind of spiritual meaning in it."

What gradual or sudden losses are you currently experiencing?

_____

_____

_____

_____

How do you feel about these losses?

_____

_____

_____

Is there an opportunity for you to create meaning from the loss? If so, how?

_____

_____

_____

_____

Happiness, Optimism, and Longevity

"I believe the second half of one's life is meant to be better than the first half. The first half is finding out how you do it. And the second half is enjoying it."

—Frances Lear

If your emotional outlook on life is an optimistic one, you increase your chances of living longer—it's a fact. One study says that people who view aging as a positive experience live an average of seven and a half years longer than those who look at it negatively, and that pessimists have a risk of death 19 percent greater than average. According to Becca Levy, a Ph.D. with the Yale School of Public Health, "The power of optimism is even greater than that of lower blood pressure or reduced cholesterol—each of which lengthens life by about four years, according to some studies."

Happy, optimistic women typically feel personal control over their lives, and those with little or no control over their lives suffer lower morale and worse health. You can't blame your unhappiness simply on aging. Social scientists interviewed representative samples of people of all ages and found that no time of life is notably happier or unhappier.

In fact, the National Opinion Research Center did a long-term survey that found that people are happier than one might expect, and happiness does not appear to depend significantly on external circumstances. Although viewing life as a tragedy has a long and honorable history, the responses of random samples of people around the world about their happiness paints a much rosier picture.

But how does one stay optimistic? Aging doesn't necessarily mean we become less happy and more pessimistic. Start by taking personal responsibility for your own happiness. Don't blame other people or external events for making you unhappy. Find what you love doing and by all means do it. Include things you enjoy in your life every day, even small things. Make a list of the positive events in your life and refer to the list when you're down. Spend five minutes every day thinking or writing about what you appreciate in life. Stay focused on the positive—even bad days have at least some bright spots.

How do you feel about this?

_____

_____

_____

_____

What can you do today, right now, to feel more optimistic about your life?

_____

_____

_____

_____

Winter Sunrise

"A day began with a fine winter sunrise, a long view of the distant horizon slowly taking on color. . . . In cities where I spent my young days, I was unaware of the power the sunrise could generate."

—Doris Grumbach, *Fifty Days of Solitude*

Today it feels like the sun never rose. It's midafternoon in February and I'm becoming more and more aware of how the lack of sunshine has me feeling miserable this winter. Maybe this is a metaphor for the "winter of my life." Just as the days grow shorter with the passing seasons, my life will become darker, less warm. I tell myself, "This thought is not a good one." I assure myself that the winter days of my life, the season of barren trees, ice on the pond, and slippery roads only mean that life will feel more vital and purposeful, and I feel better.

Each of the seasons of my life has had its meaning and reason. The spring of my life was filled with bursts of growth, weeds and all, coupled with lots of rain (tears). The summer was languid and juicy with passion. The fall of my life (which is now) is fertile with fallen leaves and the rich compost I have created that nourishes me.

So in the late fall I will tell myself that even the fading blooms are beautiful—that even as the hydrangea begins to turn its blossoms from bright white to soft brown and lavender in preparation for winter, that it is nonetheless lush with promise. I will hold the beauty of it in my eyes, bring it down into my middle to warm my bones in the winter.

I'll use the fallen, dried branches I retrieve from my lawn to kindle my fire as the signs of outer, visible growing cease for the season. I know that my growth continues unseen and that there is new life in every withered branch that clings to the tree.

How do you feel about this?

_____

_____

_____

_____

Write a metaphor describing the season of your life:

_____

_____

_____

_____

Yielding

"When two great forces collide, victory will go to the one who knows how to yield."

—Ancient Chinese philosophy

I was staying in a hotel on the beach in Puerto Rico many years back when I saw two palm trees swaying wildly in the high winds. A strong tropical storm was moving in, bending the tall trees at near right angles. Any other tree might have snapped under that kind of consistent, relentless pressure. Yet those stately palm trees were bouncing back as if nothing were happening.

The Next Fifty Years

They were yielding to the persistent force of the wind. Yielding allowed them to remain standing. And so it is with the great natural force and push of the aging process.

A close 74-year-old friend of mine once said, "We older women, we get to yield to our real feelings. If a picture is worth a thousand words, then free-flowing tears are worth a million." In addition to tears, we may find ourselves needing to yield to the sometimes difficult and challenging outset of our years. Pushing back hard against the inevitable force of nature is not nearly as powerful as yielding. The key is knowing when and how to yield, knowing how to push forward when necessary.

Of course, there are people and situations we just shouldn't yield to, like letting our teeth rot, or living with chronic pain that could be treated. We shouldn't yield to anyone who is abusive or hurtful or to any situation that makes us feel unnecessarily diminished. You will know when it is right to yield, it will feel good. It will ultimately feel growth-producing and powerful, and the victory will be yours.

How do you feel about this?

_____

_____

_____

_____

Are there some things you could choose to yield to today or that you anticipate needing to yield to in the future?

_____

_____

_____

_____

5

Our Fears

". . . you might come to realize that all your fears of getting older were unfounded, that you've been handed a much better life than you ever expected. It happens to a lot of people."

—Barbara Sher, *It's Only Too Late if You Don't Start Now: How to Create Your Second Life after 40*

Suppose Ponce de Leon really had found the fountain of eternal life? Would it have made him any happier? I don't know about him, but an AARP survey done a few years ago asked adults age 18 and older if they wanted to live to be 100. Guess what? Sixty-three percent of them said no.

Despite the fact that we have a good chance of reaching 100 (whether we like it or not) many of us fear the unknown landscape of aging. We fear illness, not having enough money, losing our mental abilities, being dependent on others, and becoming a burden to our families. Truth is, we don't have ultimate control over these situations, but we aren't completely helpless victims either. And many centenarians are still active in their communities and are practicing their skills, enjoying their hobbies, and are surprisingly healthy.

My good friend Tita Buxton (age 71) believes we shouldn't focus on what we fear about aging. "By fearing the unforeseen (aging), the future becomes what we fear"; she says this can result in a "a self-fulfilling prophecy. When I read all the stuff about aging and memory loss, I could get hung up about it rather than enjoying the life and health I do have." Tita has a point. I believe we need to face our fears and choose to live a good life in spite of them.

Remember, fear is not always bad. If you never experience it, chances are you're living too safely. You may be living beneath your capacity and avoiding challenges. The trick is to live your life fully and to do what you have to do in spite of your fear.

The worksheets that follow will assist you in examining your fears of aging, of becoming a burden, of losing control, of being in pain, of being without resources, and the ultimate fear—of death. These pages will help you face your fears honestly and realistically and help you develop a strategy for coping with them when and if they occur. The thing we cling to most fiercely is the thing that limits us the most, and until you embrace the possibility of your worst fear coming true, you can't be free from it.

"Fear—whether of life, of aging, or of change—is the worst danger you will encounter. It's the one thing that can really paralyze you."

—Sylvie Chantecaille

Fear of Aging

"October dresses in flame and gold Like a woman afraid of growing old."

—Anne Mary Lawler, poet

When we talk about our fear of growing old, what are we saying? Most of us are concerned and fearful of becoming disabled, weak, and sick. I'm not saying that some of that doesn't happen, but consider this: experts tell us that on any given day in the United States, of all our population over 65, more than 80 percent, are doing just fine physically—they're fully functional and independent.

Although our population is growing older, the rates of disability are declining. People are vigorous or healthy longer than they used to be. For example, someone 80 today may be the equivalent of a 60-year-old in the last century.

I find that if I experience each passing year as an opportunity to learn something about life, I feel more positive, more alive. In *Journey to the Heart*, author Melody Beattie says, "Now I'm learning to welcome aging, as each decade of life brings its own challenges, joys, sorrows, and teachings. . . . I don't fear aging, for I know that it's as much, and as important, a part of my life as my youth."

My 70-year-old friend Melinda once told me that one of the many things no one tells you about aging is that it is such a nice change from being young. That caused me to think about some of the "nice changes" that have occurred in recent years. I do feel more confident and a lot wiser than I did 20 years ago. In fact, lately I've been taking exercise and diet a lot more seriously and I'm feeling stronger. I also don't worry so much about what life will bring because at this point I've been through a lot, both physically and emotionally, and look!—I'm still here to talk about it.

How do you feel about this?

_____

_____

_____

_____

What are you most afraid of about aging and what can you do to help alleviate your fear?

_____

_____

_____

_____

Alone, Alive, and Worried

"Did I think more about age, aging, being and growing old when I was alone? I think so."

—Doris Grumbach, *Fifty Days of Solitude*

Maybe you're living alone right now, or you are anticipating you will be at some time in your life. Consider that you will have a choice when the time comes. Alone is a choice, *not* a condition.

Fact: People age 65 and over are adopting a living situation more commonly associated with students and young professionals—living with roommates to share companionship and expenses, and to provide some added security. These roommates, while respecting each other's independence, cook dinners for each other and provide support to one another. It's nice to know someone is there for you, and cares if you come home at night.

Consider these two scenarios:

First: You've been living safe and secure with your longtime husband in a three-bedroom home. Then he dies. You have some savings and a bit of income from Social Security plus a pension. When you add it all together, you have enough to maintain your home. After a year or two your grief subsides and you feel relatively comfortable in your home. However, each time you descend the stairs to the basement with the laundry, you worry about falling. You imagine spending a day or two with a sprained ankle just sitting on the damp basement floor until someone realizes your predicament. If you had a roommate, she would know right away if you didn't return from the laundry room. She could call 911 for you and keep you company until help arrives.

Second: You're living alone when you receive bad news by telephone concerning a dear friend. Silent and teary, you hang up the phone. Your roommate senses your despair, brings you a cup of tea, and patiently listens while you tell her what happened.

How do you feel about these two scenarios?

_____

_____

_____

_____

What alternate living choices are you willing to consider in the future?

_____

_____

_____

_____

Fear of Being a Burden

"I have a duty to all who care for me—not to be a problem, not to be a burden. I must carry my age lightly for all our sakes, and thank God I still can."

—Florida Scott-Maxwell, *The Measure of My Days*

I ponder my own future and that of my aging women friends. Some are childless and living on their own; some have children living all around the country. Who will be there for us, and do we want them to be? I'm not counting on anyone to help me with the challenges of the future, but I can't help worrying that I might someday become a burden.

Sometimes I wonder, who will be there for me when I'm an old woman? Who will monitor the doctors and ask all the right questions? Who will post notes on the refrigerator reminding me when to take my pills? Who will visit me? Who will help me stay engaged in the world? Who will listen to my fears and offer empathy?

I felt sad recently when over coffee my 68-year-old friend Mary told me, "I'm getting to know my neighbors so that someone in my building will notice if three days' worth of newspapers are piled up outside my door!" That prompted me to think. How about we all band together? I toy with the idea of communal living, of creating an enclave of like-minded women friends sometime in the future. We could be there for each other.

The way you approach life now will affect the quality of your old age and whether or not you become burdensome. Try investing in a wider world by making friends of all ages. Make sure your doctors will be there when you need them by finding doctors that are younger than you are. Spend less and save more, pay attention to nutrition, and for goodness sake, exercise more.

We are ultimately responsible for our own lives. Even so, the time may come when I'll need help. In my mind, when the time comes I will not consider myself a burden. Instead I will consider that I may need, as we all do, support and encouragement. I promise to get myself one of those emergency alert buzzers when I get to a certain age. I wonder when will that be?

How do you feel about this?

_____

_____

What life decisions can you make now that will affect future challenges?

_____

_____

_____

_____

Fear of Pain

"Growing older is not something to be glorified but neither is it to be feared; there is loss and pain in aging . . . but also laughter and wisdom."

—Susan Feldman, et al., *Something That Happens to Other People: Stories of Women Growing Older*

There are two categories of physical pain—chronic and temporary. At different points in our lives we will be confronted by either or both. A wide range of studies have shown that women tend to feel acute pain more intensely than men do. They are also more vulnerable to a variety of painful conditions that include migraines, arthritis, fibromyalgia, pelvic pain, and abdominal pain of various kinds. Men and women both suffer back pain equally. Perhaps it's more acceptable to women to talk about their pain. Whatever the case, fear makes pain less tolerable.

Of all symptoms, pain is probably the most terrifying, to patients as well as to doctors. But few doctors are actually trained to deal with it. Now there is a special breed of doctors called pain specialists who see pain not as incidental to disease, but as a disease in its own right. Today, most major hospitals have a pain management team. In addition, our choices for treating pain are wide and varied. Not long ago, the idea of treating pain with acupuncture, hypnosis, or biofeedback would have raised many an eyebrow within the medical mainstream.

As you mature, you are bound to run up against increased pain or discomfort from surgery, arthritis, muscle aches, etc. Your fear about pain creates even more discomfort. If you become tense or fretful about your condition, the pain increases. The pain also increases if you are uninformed and fretful as a result.

When people prepare for surgery they have less pain and fewer complications and they heal faster. Preparation includes gathering honest, clear, straightforward information. I was extremely grateful when my surgeon said I would experience pain after my gallbladder operation. She said that acute pain for a period of time was normal and that it would be well managed with medication. During my overnight hospital stay, her honest words came back to me and helped me to experience less stress, in turn helping me cope with the intense discomfort. Stress creates more pain, but the pain itself is going to create stress. It can become a vicious cycle.

In addition to your doctor's honest information, one of the ways to break the stress/pain cycle is to learn how to meditate. Ask your doctor about meditation classes or buy a relevant book or relaxation tape. When it comes to surgery, for instance, start practicing the technique so that by the time you get to the operating room, you've become a master. After practice you will be able to lie there, elicit the relaxation response, and feel a lot better.

One of my favorite pain management techniques is visualization. I imagine I'm on the island of Kauai in Hawaii when I have dental work done. Also known as guided imagery, this technique involves using your mind's eye to picture something that will both distract your thoughts and promote a sense of release and relaxation.

So if as you age you are fearful of pain, remember there are ways to manage it. As women we need to fight, if necessary, to make our doctors listen. We are not hysterical because we cry when we are in pain. We need to demand respect and receive it, but first we need to respect ourselves; ask for what you need, seek information about what you don't know, and most of all accept that pain is part of life and there are things you can do to comfort yourself to reduce your fear.

How do you feel about this?

_____

_____

_____

_____

The Next Fifty Years

Are you in physical pain and what can you do to manage it?

_____

_____

_____

_____

Fear of Losing Control

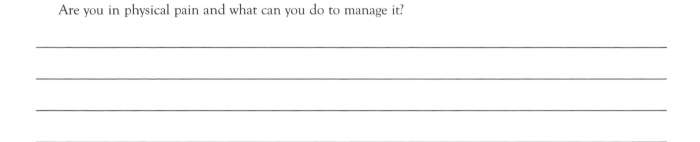

"We think we know what's going on, that we have control of our lives; we make plans, have date books and schedules, and then we turn around to see ourselves and realize our lives have their own composition, their own movement."

—Natalie Goldberg, *Long Quiet Highway*

Riding back from the library on a beautiful late March afternoon, feeling the beginnings of spring, I was met head-on at a stoplight by a speeding, out-of-control, four-wheel-drive, teenage-driven vehicle. It was just one week after I had signed the contract for my first book entitled *I Wasn't Ready to Say Goodbye*. The book deals with sudden death. There I was dealing with the possibility of my own. The windows were rolled down to let in the sun and air, the back seat was stacked with library books on death. The impact of the speeding vehicle caused me to experience extreme whiplash. I was immediately disoriented and dizzy. The police arrived within seconds, just as I was trying to call 911 on my cell phone. Amazing how difficult it is to remember those three easy numbers when your brain has banged against the inside of your skull.

One minute I was a newly contracted, soon-to-be author, gainfully employed psychotherapist, and part-time consultant—the next minute I was suffering a traumatic, closed-head brain injury. That afternoon I was in control of my life and the pursuit of happiness. The next day I was dependent on others to make decisions for me, to drive for me, to think logically for me, to help me walk straight and find words, to guide me from room to room when I got lost in my own house.

I called my office and in a halting, kindergarten voice explained that I'd been in a car accident, I wasn't able to come in, that maybe it would take a week or so to recover. That source of income ended when it took two and half years to recover. Most of the first year I felt and acted like I was 80 years old or more. I had to walk with a cane so I wouldn't bang into walls. My neuropsychologist said this was normal. Not for *me* it wasn't! I was a hustler, a juggler of many balls in the air. Now I was having trouble making toast and remembering the word for milk (I called it "white stuff"). Now I was taking a shower only to forget which comes first, shampoo or conditioner. Did I remember to wash all my parts or did I forget under my arms again?

I used to be in control of my life. I knew exactly what the plan was and where I was going. Before the accident rearranged my life, I was going to spend every Friday, all day, just working on the book. I would see my therapy clients all day Thursdays, and after four o'clock on Monday, Tuesday, and Wednesday when I got back from my consulting/office manager job. The schedule was suddenly different now, life going slower than I could have ever imagined, taking on its own composition, its own movement.

Once I could remember some words and start typing again (thank God for spell check) I found myself with endless hours to work on my book, to sit in the garden (even though I couldn't garden), to read for short periods, to be with my grandson and children in ways I'd never had time for in the past. When I began to give up total control of my recovery, I began to feel better.

I'm reminded of what Barbara Sher said in her book, *It's Only Too Late if You Don't Start Now:* "When you give up your youthful urgency to control every outcome, you can finally throw yourself wholeheartedly, without conflict, into whatever matters to you." I was deepening, digging into new soil, accessing my "new brain," trying on another self, becoming a me I had not known before, and the control—the controller, the higher power—was driving this time.

Acknowledge that you have no control over outside events. Whatever success you enjoyed at work, whatever plans you made for the future, gave you the illusion you had mastered the world and taken control of your own life. Brushes with death or sudden life changes can help us develop an increased awareness of how little we really control. Life goes on making its own plans, producing its own troubles and joys. This awareness of how little we control and the shortness of time isn't all negative; it also gives us an increased freedom. We are given a chance to become less tyrannized by worry about what other people might think, by a need to be liked, and less tyrannized by death itself.

The Next Fifty Years

How do you feel about this?

_____

_____

_____

_____

In what way has life shown you that you are not totally in control?

_____

_____

_____

_____

Oh No, Not Public Transportation!

"It's important as we age to take into account that there will be certain realities that should be faced squarely and realistically. One of these is driving."

—Tita Buxton, 71

My husband, Steve, and I have been traveling by car to the most northerly coast of Maine for many years to a house where we spend two weeks every year. As we grow older, I'm imagining a time when we'll need to fly to Maine instead of drive. We would then need to rent a car and drive the 45 minutes to the house where we stay. I've thought, one day we won't be able to do even that much driving. Am I sad about that prospect? You bet!

Driving is synonymous with independence and freedom. Never mind driving 900 miles to Maine, driving plays such a key role in daily life, it's no surprise that an individual's physical and mental health may suffer when driving ceases and outside activities dwindle. Surrendering the car keys may be emotionally traumatic and lead to depression and physical or cognitive declines. Transportation is the glue that holds life together. The freedom to come and go as we want, when we want, is ultimately a personal responsibility. We need to ask ourselves the hard questions of where we would live and how we would get around if we couldn't access some form of transportation. Some rural or suburban areas have sparse public transportation and a lack of nearby goods and services.

My 71-year-old friend Tita says, "As sight and reaction time diminish, we need to think of other ways of getting around other than driving ourselves. We need to take into account other people's lives that we might be endangering. Difficult as it is, we can ask others (usually younger) who might be able to drive us places. We must think of these kinds of alternatives."

I think most of us mature, evolved women are willing to self-regulate ourselves by restricting our driving under certain conditions: bad weather, highways at night, heavy traffic, unfamiliar areas, rush hour, or long distances. Self-regulation is a gradual process, not a sudden shift in behavior. Over time you will develop conscious strategies to compensate for failing vision, slower reflexes, and stiffer joints. Chronic illnesses and multiple medications also make driving more stressful.

Should you hang up your keys? An article in *AARP the Magazine* suggests you ask yourself these questions:

- Do you find yourself saying, "Whew, that was close"?
- Do cars seem to appear from nowhere?
- At intersections, do cars proceed when you feel you have the right of way?
- Are gaps in traffic harder to judge?
- Do others honk at you?
- After driving, do you feel physically exhausted?
- Do you think you are slower than you used to be in reacting to dangerous driving situations?
- Are family members or friends afraid to be a passenger when you drive?
- Do intersections bother you because there is so much to watch for in all directions?
- Have you had an increased number of near accidents in the last year?

When you shop for a car in your later years, look for options like automatic transmissions, power brakes and steering, automatic windows, and seat adjustments and mirrors that will help you compensate for diminished flexibility or strength. By all means, get regular vision and hearing checkups. As you get older, get used to public transportation while you still drive so it won't be so hard on you later on. Contact your local agency on aging. They may have a program that helps seniors become more familiar with public transportation and other options.

Health combined with age is a more important predictor of driver self-regulation than age alone. So if you're an 85-year-old woman with good vision, good reaction times, and good health, keep on driving. In fact, the Insurance Institute for Highway Safety says older drivers are less likely than teenagers to hurt people in car accidents. But get your eyes checked at least once a year and make sure your ears are working too. You don't want to mistake honking horns for migrating geese.

How do you feel about this?

What transportation alternatives are you willing to consider when the time comes?

Fear of Dying

"I guess I probably don't have that much longer on this Earth, but I may as well make the best of it."

—Sarah L. Delany, *On My Own at 107*

When you think hard on it, are you afraid of dying or are you afraid that you haven't given your all to life? I'm not so much afraid of dying as I am of not having *lived*. I've faced death in a real way—a head-on car crash, a near drowning on the Salt River in Arizona, a plane that nearly plummeted to earth in a snowstorm, and a terrifying episode in civil-war-torn Mozambique in the 1980s where my husband and I faced the danger of a deadly ambush. I have had to confront my fear of dying. In the process, I've become less afraid of solitude and I've discovered a new self-confidence. All the conventional limitations that used to constrict my behavior have fallen away.

When faced with our own mortality, we may begin to question other aspects of our lives, including the choices we have made along the way. Alongside our fear of dying, questions may arise such as: Did I chose the right partner? The most fulfilling career path? Am I happy with my current life and do I have the courage to change before I no longer have options? It's those little things left undone that came to mind as I was facing death. I thought about the book I hadn't written that I had intended to write "one of these days." I was sorry that I hadn't told my husband, children, and friends often enough how much I loved them.

The distinction between a life worth leaving and one worth living is probably different for each of us. For some of us, death will be a kind friend and a release from pain. In *Soulwork*, BettyClare Moffatt says death will be a "release into the all-embracing light, as a reward, not a punishment." That works for me.

If it's worth seeing or hearing or doing, I'm doing it now so death will seem less frightening. It's hard to use your available time with all your heart until you've eyed death on the road up ahead. These days I'm trying hard not to put off, hold back, or save anything that would add laughter and radiance to my life and the lives of those I love. Every morning when I open my eyes, I tell myself that this day is special. Every day, every minute, every breath truly is a gift from God.

How do you feel about this?

_____

_____

_____

_____

What can you do now that you've been putting off?

_____

_____

Fear of Abuse

"The stereotype of aging as a progressive loss of function is generally true only for people who stop functioning."

—Joan Borysenko, *A Woman's Book of Life*

Recent studies suggest that 4 percent of seniors, more than one million Americans over 65, may be physically abused or neglected each year. These victims are often frightened and confused. Frequently, the abuser and abused reside together. Many are dependent on their abusers for daily care. Issues of power and control are at the core of this abuse.

Some older women find themselves in situations where they need assistance with life tasks. Perhaps they feel powerless and afraid. It is women in these circumstances who are often hesitant to bring abuse to the attention of those in a position to help. You need not allow someone to abuse or mistreat you just because you are older and in need of assistance. There are professionals who can help, should you find yourself in this situation.

No matter what age you are, domestic abuse can take on many forms. Mistreatment ranges from physical and psychological abuse to passive and active neglect. The abuse may include the exploitation of financial resources. It can also take the form of coercive behaviors such as progressive social isolation, deprivation, and intimidation; psychological, emotional, sexual, or verbal abuse of a person by a past or present intimate partner.

It is important to speak with someone who can help you. In all cases, it is essential that authorities be notified immediately—adult protective services, elder abuse, victims' assistance services. Let someone know. Talk to your physician, clergy person, nurse, health aide, dentist, optometrist, or other professional healthcare provider. These health professionals recognize that they may be the only ones in a position of trust and confidence to identify and report the abuse. Remember, your respect, dignity, and maybe even your life are at stake.

How do you feel about this?

_____

_____

_____

_____

What action will you take on your behalf should you feel abused?

_____

_____

_____

_____

Fear of Being a Bag Lady

"[It] takes so much effort to hold on to the illusion of youth, to keep the fear of age at bay."

—Betty Friedan

When my aging friends and I get together, inevitably one of them brings up the fear of not having enough financial resources to make old age a positive experience.

I ask them, how much do you need? Realistically, how much money do we need to be happy, to feel secure? Do you think you'll be living in the street at some point in your older years? (See "Living Well on Less" in chapter 15.)

Let's look at the reality: economizing can have the effect of forcing us to think creatively about our lifestyle and our priorities, to reflect on what matters to us. Looking for ways to enjoy life while reducing the amount of money we spend builds character. It's not a disgrace.

You don't have to deplete your current resources if you begin to live creatively and actively seek out alternatives to spending more than you can afford to. For instance, take advantage of senior discounts, offer personal services instead of giving expensive gifts, read books from the library instead of buying them, and discover the pleasures that can come from a walk in a beautiful place instead of shopping at the mall.

If you're worried about resources, who says you can't work forever if you want and need to? Why spend one-fifth to one-third of your life in retirement? Along with millions of other women, we are likely to be healthy and active well into our futures, so why not make some money while we're at it?

Most of all, try not to live in fear. Living in fear is not really living.

How do you feel about this?

_____

_____

_____

_____

Name some practical and creative ways you could economize, starting today:

_____

_____

_____

_____

Fear of Asking for Help

"There are some things only we can do for our emotional, physical and spiritual health. . . . Yet there are needs we cannot take care of alone."

—Amy E. Dean, *Night Light*

When I was suffering from the acute stages of a mild traumatic brain injury in my late forties, under doctor's orders, I couldn't drive for almost two years. I had the reaction time, visual depth of field, and driving ability of a 90-year-old. I *needed* the help of friends and family and, for the first time in my life, I *had* to ask for help. It was a painful lesson for militantly independent me.

Doing nice things for others may be appreciated and even earn you a reputation as being likable. But did you know that allowing others to do things for you will also make them like you? It makes people feel good to help others.

Many of us have been taught that we shouldn't admit to our pain and suffering, so we bear them in silence. We begin to feel alone, yet if we need companionship, we need companionship. And we need to ask for what we need.

Here are some suggestions: If you live alone and/or need help from time to time, organize a support system of friends, relatives, and organizations that you can call on. In addition, make sure that your home is organized so that a helpful neighbor or friend can find what is needed to give you a hand with medications or special instructions. Make sure important names and phone numbers are handy and visible for all to see.

My dear friend Tita (71 years old) recently told me, "In our society people have learned that you shouldn't ask for help. Was that in early elementary school where students are 'supposed' to think for themselves—that each should be an independent thinker? Well, it certainly doesn't help when we're older." She said that in her view, asking someone for help is a positive, not a negative, and that some things are even more fun when done with the support of someone else. Don't be afraid to ask for help when you need it. You may even like it.

How do you feel about this?

_____

_____

_____

_____

If you had to ask someone for help, who would it be? Why?

_____

_____

_____

_____

Fear of the Future

"Planning what I can for the future is responsible of me, then I return to the now. To truly live a life that's mine, to create a life of my own choosing, I have to show up in the present, not stay lost in the past or be transported into the future."

—Janet F. Quinn, *I Am a Woman Finding My Voice*

Some days I fear taking on the responsibility of planning for my future. I know I should prepare, but what if I make a mistake in the planning? What if I don't account for the fact that I will die on Tuesday at 1:18 P.M. in August of 2030? Suppose I make plans for my future and then don't show up for them because I became senile instead? Suppose I forget who I made the plan for? My sister Marilyn and her husband cashed in their savings, including their IRA, bought their dream house, and he died six months later. Boom. Up and left her holding "the plan."

According to Harold Bloomfield in his provocative book entitled *Making Peace with Your Past: The Six Essential Steps to Enjoying a Great Future,* "The three most profound questions in every person's life are: Who am I? Where did I come from? Where am I going?" The root cause of human suffering, he says, is "the accumulation of unprocessed experience from the past." I say it's the accumulation of too many plans that might not come true.

I believe that women who learn to adapt, who learn to create opportunities and accept their limitations, will have a better quality of life. Women who make choices that will allow them to spend more time doing what they want to do and who have some kind of game plan, or goal, will ultimately age more successfully.

So I plan to sit down and ask myself, "Where did I come from?" I will need to answer this before I can ask myself, "Who am I?" Then I will start the honest assessment of where I am going with my life.

How do you feel about this? Are you fearful of the future?

_____

_____

_____

_____

If you were less fearful, what would your life be like?

_____

_____

_____

_____

6

Our Love Lives and Relationships

"Love comes to those who still hope although they've been disappointed—to those who still believe although they've been betrayed, to those who still need to love although they've been hurt before, and to those who have the courage and faith to build trust again."

Anonymous, from the Internet

American women don't give up easily when pursuing happiness. They marry, divorce, and marry again. Women who grew up in the feminist era demand fairness. For many, the loss of a partner represents a respite from household drudgery and a life of serving others. Why hook up with another taker? They were willing to get the "one" and have kids, and then stopped being interested in the male sex in general.

I know many women in their fifties who are not attractive, but they've got *joie de vivre*. They have bounce; they have vitality. That's what attracts men. Charm has nothing to do with looks. These women don't take themselves too seriously and they know how to laugh. They don't go around moaning and groaning.

Most of our mothers lived restricted sex lives. They looked much older at our age than we do. Fear of expressing sexual desire helped to age our parents because of all the stipulations and anxieties on sexual freedoms. The major fears women have had are due to rules set by men on what women should and can be sexually. The truth is, many men just can't keep pace sexually with women. Even if we senior women haven't tried all the positions in the *Kama Sutra*, we know we are nonetheless real women in many different areas of our lives.

We grow old and we think we're no longer lovable. Why? Because our skin doesn't fit as well, or the bounce is gone? Can an 80-year-old woman have good sex? Absolutely. She might not be doing acrobatics, but she can enjoy sex, she can enjoy the intimacy, she can even have orgasms. Health, medication, and hormonal changes, including declining testosterone, have an impact on a woman's sexuality, as does your attitude about aging. But sex can be enjoyed throughout life.

Alongside the younger ones, we older women have a choice of "lovestyle" also. More and more people are opting to live together rather than marry. Cohabitation without the benefit of marriage is especially favored by older persons who want to protect their separate financial lives, including the right to collect Social Security benefits.

In *Women Who Love Too Much*, Robin Norwood says, "When being in love means being in pain we are loving too much. When most of our conversations with intimate friends are about him, his problems, his thoughts, his feelings—and nearly all our sentences begin with 'he . . . ,' we are loving too much." Women have discovered that putting their entire focus on their mates created an imbalance in the relationship. Many are reassessing their long-term marriages and are challenging their mates to be more sensitive to their needs. Women are finding their voice in relationships more than they ever have in the past. And if their partners won't hear them and respond accordingly, they are opting out.

Sharing the experience of aging with a husband or lover may not be in the cards for every woman, and it becomes important to seek out safe human touch like hugs or therapeutic massage. As we age, we need to approach our sex lives with honesty and a willingness to learn about our changing bodies. Talk about honesty, an AARP survey revealed that 50 percent of women would choose chocolate over making love.

For most women over 50, married or single, questions about love relationships, old or new, continue to arise. This chapter will ask you to consider some of the situations inherent in divorce and dating after 50, like learning to trust oneself in relationship. The subjects of living within the challenges of a long-term marriage and marrying again after 50 are briefly explored, as are the tough issues associated with the death or illness of a husband or lover. Every one of the following essays could, of course, be a book on the topic of love and romance. As with the other sections, take your time to respond to the questions and skip those essays that don't apply to you.

Get Hugged!

"When you hug someone you love, take hold of the person and in the first breath, breathe in and out, be totally present."

—Thich Nhat Hanh

Researchers tell us that we all need four hugs a day. The touch of another human being is a necessity. Human touch actually activates many biological mechanisms that help the body heal itself.

I read about a university project that trained older volunteers to massage premature, drug-exposed, failure-to-thrive newborns. The researchers were sure the infants would experience some beneficial effects because in some earlier studies, massage therapy had resulted in decreased levels of stress and increased physical and cognitive gains. But in the study, something else happened as well: the massagers also started to benefit. They started having more contact with friends, drank less coffee, and suffered less depression. This study shows that whether people are touching or being touched, they not only feel better, they *are* better.

Hugging, snuggling, petting, stroking, and touching are good for your health, your heart, and your relationships. It can even become habit-forming. It seems a terrible shame that such a wonderful resource is often limited to times of grief and sexual encounters. Hugging and being hugged can do a great deal to improve the quality of your everyday life. No matter your age, it feeds a very basic human need. Ruth Beckford, the author of *Still Groovin'*, says that "a hug is a gourmet meal to my skin."

But what happens if you live alone? How do you get your hugs then? My husband travels a great deal for his job, sometimes weeks at a time. I turn to my cats for petting. After all, their role in life is to be petted, touched, and stroked. I also turn to my grown daughter (who lives nearby) and grandson for hugs, as well as several close friends.

To add to the mix, I purchased several small down-filled comforters. I keep one in the living room for watching TV and one in the bedroom for afternoon naps. Kids know how to get their nurturing needs met—they get attached to their blankets, dolls, and teddy bears. From observing how children get their "hug" needs met, I've decided to wear furry coats (feels like a teddy bear) and scatter velvety soft pillows around my house to hug. I even

Our Love Lives and Relationships

invested in a velvet couch. In the colder months I wear as many cashmere sweaters and fleece tops as I can afford. Other surrogate huggers include cozy slippers, cups of tea, and warm, sudsy bubble baths.

What can you do to get your four human hugs each day?

_____

_____

_____

_____

What "hug surrogates" can you bring into your life?

_____

_____

_____

_____

Expressing Your Sexual Self

"I'm intending to walk around town as a sexy old lady, the kind that no Boy Scout need hurry to help cross the street."

—Judith Viorst, *Forever Fifty*

You know what's upsetting? Those messages from the media and society at large that an older women shouldn't be too sexy or too vigorous or too interested in life, that it's not ladylike. Part of our problem is that many of us still see ourselves the way we saw our grandmothers—sexless and frail. We need to fight that societal stereotyping. Sex is not just for the young. There are few reasons that men and women can't have active, fulfilling sex lives into their nineties. In fact, some women become more orgasmic in their later years.

We baby boomer women came of age believing we had a right to sexual pleasure, and that belief is not about to evaporate at age 65 or 75. Even so, some of us are just as happy without sex. Close ties with friends and family are as important to quality of life as sex is for some women. Of course, getting older does bring certain physical changes that can cause problems, but fortunately those problems can usually be treated.

There's a difference between being sexy and having sex—one is an attitude and the other is a physical act. The image of the older woman as sexless needs some rethinking. I know plenty of "sexy" older women. Perhaps you're one of them. While sags and bulges don't necessarily symbolize sex as well as firm young skin does, there are more intrinsic qualities that create the sexual chemistry that attracts us to each other. Sex is not just as it is portrayed in the movies—sweaty and crazy. It's a lot more than that and it's defined by our stage in life. It's an expression of our connection to our partner and connection to ourselves. If you choose to and you're interested, you can be sexual until you die.

The good news is that sex does change as we age. For instance, around 50, men tend to become more emotional about lovemaking, and they start seeking more closeness and intimacy. Women, on the other hand, become more independent and assertive. Even so, some women don't understand that their partners will need more foreplay and a little more understanding during sex. On the other hand, you may resent having to give more at this point in your life. If you've been harboring resentment over issues you haven't confronted as a couple, you may not be willing give more.

Did you know that many men have the same strong feelings about aging as women do—the fears, the anxiety—and they're just as self-conscious about their pot bellies as you may be about the fat on your thighs? There are some steps you can take to feel good about yourself if you're just beginning a sexual relationship. Until you feel secure with the man you're sexually involved with, you can hide your sagging arms with sleeves. You don't have to wear a short nightgown if your knees are knobby. After a while, when you're feeling confident in the relationship and feeling better about your older body, strut around the bedroom nude if you want to with your head held high. Self-acceptance is sexy. Also, people who work out feel better about their bodies, plus working out releases brain chemicals that make you feel energetic and happy.

Life circumstances can get in the way of a fulfilling sex life. At this age you may find yourself in either an empty nest or an overpopulated one where an older child has returned home, or in-laws and elderly parents are living with you.

After 50, looks are less important than intelligence, a sense of humor, and a sense of style. Sex in a committed relationship is important—but more important for men than for women. Over age 50, the quality of sex depends much more on the overall quality of a relationship than it does for young couples.

Frequent sex may help you live longer. Sex burns calories, works muscles, and boosts the body's immune system. Sex can even relieve pain by releasing endorphins and producing cortisone. Vaginal lubrication is less of problem for women over 60 who regularly have sex or masturbate.

A study of 18- to 101-year-olds showed that a good sex life can make you look younger as well as feel younger. The persons who reported having the best sex lives looked four to seven years younger than their real age. Good sex helps both physical and mental health by reducing stress, providing relaxation, and enhancing contentment.

Can sex get better with age? Absolutely. There's more physical pleasure, more free time, no concern about pregnancy, no children at home (hopefully). People accept their bodies, they experiment, they understand their desires—sex becomes more than a mad, furious rush to perform the act. For couples who understand it, the slowing of sexual response can be an advantage. They tend to get more in sync. Bad sex won't become good sex simply because you're older. But it can be great sex if you communicate with your partner, and if you learn that intimacy means there are no questions you should ever be afraid to ask.

Not everyone over 50 chooses to or can have sex. Perhaps you have a long history of lack of interest in or fear of sexual intercourse; or the desire is there but there's no opportunity to meet a potential sexual partner. No matter what the cause, countless older couples are living happy, contented lives without sex. As we age, we need access to a larger physical repertoire such as touching, caressing, kissing, and other expressions of physical affection. As our bodies change, so too do the ways that help us feel good.

The hormonal shifts of menopause can have an effect on one's sex life. Like a lot of women, when menopause arrived, my interest in sex left but after a while my desire came back. A substantial body of research has exploded decades of mythology about female sexuality. Libido requires a good supply of testosterone in women as well as in men, and there is a testosterone cream that women can use to help with libido. Don't be afraid to discuss issues in your sex life with your doctor or gynecologist. In fact, you may have to initiate the discussion; your doctor may not bring up this touchy subject, because many medical professionals still don't think of older people as sexual beings.

AIDS cases are rising more than twice as fast among older persons as young adults. You undoubtedly realize that anyone who has unprotected sex is taking a risk. But did you know that more than 13 percent of Americans who have AIDS are over age 50? Divorcees and widows who are reentering the dating scene after a long hiatus may be especially at risk.

In our older years, sexual desire doesn't just happen. Most women have to be physically stimulated to feel desire for their partner. Ironically, this means that women who think they need to be in the mood to have sex might in fact need to have sex to get in the mood. To rekindle desire, treat sex as play and exhibit your sensual personality. As Mae West said when she was in her mid-eighties, "When you've got the personality, you don't need the nudity." Use hugs, kisses, and gentle caresses to show tenderness. Emotional rewards can be as fulfilling as physical ones. Be creative. Planting a garden, baking bread, building a piece of furniture—or any creative activity—can rev up your sex drive.

Women who have enjoyed sex in the past will likely continue to do so. Single women have told me that when they want sex, they have it with themselves. Women need to know that they can take care of their sexual needs. Even if you don't have a man in your life, you are still a sexual being.

How do you feel about your sex life?

_____

_____

_____

_____

Are there ways you could make it better?

_____

_____

_____

_____

When Husbands Die

*Staring at my ceiling,
counting dreams of you at midnight . . .*

—Marilyn Houston, writer and poet

In *Evenings at Five*, Gail Godwin writes, "It was so quiet after he was gone; there was no music, and that voice wasn't there." As I read that passage I felt a stinging sadness. Although I deeply crave solitude and quiet, the absence of sound would be the hardest part of losing my husband.

Acceptance is difficult. A client named Andrea recalled the night after her husband's funeral: "I couldn't sleep, so I spent half the night cleaning the kitchen. I said the word 'widow' out loud to myself, tasting its bitter sound in my mouth. Even though I'd been preparing to say this word for the two years since his leukemia was diagnosed, it was still a challenge to say it." Brenda, a 61-year-old client, told me that for the first year and a half after her husband died, she couldn't concentrate enough to read a full paragraph at one sitting. "I couldn't focus. When someone you love dies, a part of you dies too. It's almost three years now, and I feel as if I am just now beginning to think."

A good 50 percent of women over the age of 65 are widows. About 85 percent of wives outlive their husbands. There are literally millions of women who no longer have husbands, yet most of them are doing quite well. In fact, women do better on their own then men do. Author Riane Eisler once said, "I was without a partner for ten years, and I have good friends who are without partners, and they do just fine."

Grieving is the hardest work you will ever do. Even though you may spend years caring for a chronically ill husband, you may be emotionally unequipped for his death. When the final event happens, we are rarely, if ever, ready. We hope for a miracle.

Although loss of a spouse is one of the most stressful life events one can experience, in the long term, most older women find that widowhood is accompanied by a positive shift into a new life phase. They want to take back control of their lives, test out skills they learned over a lifetime, exercise new feelings of strength and self-confidence that maturity can bring. Marcel Proust once said that "happiness is good for the body, but it is grief which develops strengths of mind."

The death of your husband, as hard as it is to think about, can ultimately

100

The Next Fifty Years

present an opportunity for great learning—to do things one never did before. My friend Barbara told me, "My husband's death was, and continues to be, the most defining moment in my life. I'm the same person I was before but now I know who I am."

Many women begin to enjoy their single life as soon as the sharp edges of grief have worn off. Seventy-two-year-old Liz related her story. "My husband died of a heart attack. We were married for 41 years and he was my first love. I'm still lonely at times, but I've made some new single friends, which is nice. I'm starting to enjoy life again."

There is a danger in adopting grief as a way of life. If you do, you're still making your husband responsible for your well-being. Another danger lies in putting your deceased husband on a pedestal, which makes it easy to remember only the good, so that going forward, no one else can measure up. You may be using this view as an excuse to prevent yourself from renewing your life and loving another person. Not everyone who is bereaved will experience the same things. The key task is to accept the reality of the death, experience the pain of grief, adjust to life without the deceased, and memorialize the loved one in order to move on.

Natalie Goldberg in *Long Quiet Highway* says, "Whether we know it or not, we transmit the presence of everyone we have ever known, as though by being in each other's presence we exchange our cells, pass on some of our life force, and then we go on carrying that other person in our body, not unlike springtime when certain plants in fields we walk through attach their seeds in the form of small burrs to our socks, our pants, our caps. . . . This is how we survive long after we are dead."

The word "widow" comes from the Sanskrit and means "empty." But does it have to be an empty time, or can one still fill up on what life has to offer? What are your thoughts and feelings about this?

_____

_____

_____

_____

_____

Long Married

". . . the later years can also be a time of renewed bonds and greater understanding—a time when your marriage grows stronger and more intimate, more rewarding than ever before."

—Steve Brody, Ph.D., and Cathy Brody, M.S., *Renew Your Marriage at Midlife*

Growth is possible in long-term marriage, more so than in a life dedicated solely to oneself. It is also possible to avoid finding out who you are by hiding out in the marriage and by subscribing everything to your spouse. If you've been married a long time, it's important to ask yourself, "Am I still growing in my marriage or am I hiding out there?"

You may be revving up at this time in your life (children grown, nest empty, postmenopausal zest), and your husband may be winding down and readying for retirement. Developmental needs and life-cycle changes are the tectonic plates of our emotional lives. They move deep underground, outside of our control, responding to different pressures. Conflicts in long-term marriages are not always what they seem. First you need to assess whether conflicts are actually time-of-life differences or chronic relationship patterns rearing their head anew.

It's impossible to live in a long-term relationship without losing patience, without conflict, and without being thoughtless from time to time. We are human after all.

Fran Sumner, 95 and author of *The Love Affair of Fran and Maurie*, was married for 67 years. Her advice: "Be careful of each other's feelings." If the love you have for your partner is strong and you have a history of practicing kindness and generosity with each other, you are probably more likely to prioritize those values within your relationship. You may discover you would rather be together than get your own way. This can help you move past an impasse to more loving and productive negotiations.

Think of the learning and adjusting that's already gone into your long-

The Next Fifty Years

term marriage. As you age into retirement, you may find that you now have even more time to discover one another's gifts, explore mutual interests, enroll in courses together, take up a new sport together, making each other a priority.

The changes in your lives that come with age can disrupt the delicate balance of a marriage. For instance, one of you gets sick and the other now has to switch roles, or one or both of you retire and are spending a lot of time together, or the nest is finally empty. This is when the marriage must be redefined. Be open with your spouse about body changes, fluctuating weight, and self-image. Marriages that negotiate and navigate these physical and emotional challenges inevitably come out stronger.

I've been married to my husband for 21 years. We've been through challenging times, but we've managed to keep the romance alive. Here are some of my personal suggestions:

- Nurture each other's sense of humor and play.
- Write love notes to him and leave them in unexpected places.
- Give *him* flowers for no good reason.
- Tell him you want to go "out on a date."
- Send a greeting card to him at the office (or to the house if he's retired).
- Get up early one day and surprise him with breakfast and the sports page.
- Go with him to the doctor.
- Point out those things you appreciate him doing.

After reading this list to my friend Deb she suggested adding, "Let him have the TV remote once in a while!"

How do you feel about your long-term marriage?

_____

_____

_____

_____

In what ways are you willing to learn and grow in your marriage?

_____

_____

When the One You Love Is Ill

"After my husband's heart attack I was coping, but then I felt overwhelmed by strong feelings of grief. My husband was alive, so how come I was feeling such grief and loss? The answer is, our life together had changed forever."

—Susan, age 64

Older couples who have successfully negotiated the early stages of retirement may find themselves facing crises when illness upsets the longtime balance of roles and responsibilities in their relationship. We mourn our old innocent ways and our lost certainties. We face changes in lifestyle, financial security, retirement, and our spouse's physical capabilities. Perhaps over the years you developed a certain sense of security and now the rules have changed. The upside is that a brush with mortality can reorder a couple's priorities for the better. A health crisis can pull some couples apart, intensifying existing conflicts. For others, the crisis provides an opportunity for enriching the relationship.

Millions of older American women are caring for a chronically ill husband. This stressful endeavor can be hazardous to the caregiver's health, especially in cases where the chronic disease is severe. Some caregivers begin to neglect themselves and unknowingly create stress-induced health issues. To maintain your role as a functional caretaker, you must pay attention to your own needs. Taking care of yourself helps you come to terms with this life-changing crisis.

Take charge of your life and don't let your loved one's illness or disability always take center stage. Honor yourself—you're doing a very hard job and you deserve some quality time, just for you. When someone offers to lend a hand, accept their offer. Learn as much as you can about your loved one's condition, promote your loved one's independence, grieve your losses, and allow yourself to dream new dreams.

There is great strength in knowing you are not alone, so seek support from other caregivers. Check with your local hospital to see if they have caregiver support groups. You will also feel less fearful if you can involve the whole family. At weekly problem solving meetings, ask each person to describe his greatest concerns. Then discuss them. If your children are grown and living elsewhere, performing this exercise even once during a visit can break the tension and be extremely helpful.

If you are grieving over the loss of your former life with your husband, honest discussion of the changes in your relationship can ease the pain. Remember that your combined grief is both a process that make take some time, and an opportunity for deepening your marriage.

How do you feel about this?

_____

_____

_____

_____

_____

_____

_____

Divorce after 50

"Divorce after 50 presents some problems and some special blessings. . . . All of our cumulative experience gives us an advantage in divorce. . . . You have a lot of treasure to draw from."

—Micki McWade, *Daily Meditations for Surviving a Breakup, Separation, or Divorce*

Overall, we are a generation of women who have redefined life. Although some of us have never married, others have been married and divorced a number of times or have been separated for so long it feels like divorce. The divorce rate for 50-year-old women is at about 24 percent. For some women, divorce at this stage in their lives is about freedom that offers a sense of liberation from a subservient role. For others, especially those who haven't chosen it, divorce creates anxiety and extreme fear.

Before you make the decision to divorce, it's important to be realistic. Ask yourself if you'll be happier alone. I've had clients who left their marriages believing they would find Mr. Right, and although some did, some also found their relationship with the new man was every bit as problematic. Make sure you're not thinking you'd be happier with someone else.

How bad does a marriage have to be before getting out is the only answer? How much potential good remains to make it worth working through all the problems? Let's say you've worked to resolve the problems in your relationship and have tried to accept things the way they are. But you're still struggling with what might be best for you—stay or leave. If you stay when you should be getting out, you risk emotional death, and your relationship will die if you continue to obsess about leaving.

It is an inescapable truth that some marriages cannot and should not be saved. Everyone understands there's such a thing as being in a relationship with someone who is so bossy, controlling, domineering, overwhelming, and destructive that you have to get out. Patterns of toxic marital interaction keep the body in a state of unhealthy physical arousal. They create a psychological climate of helplessness where neither spouse can surmount the hostility and negativity that has seeped into almost every marital interaction.

Some of the women I spoke to simply said they wanted the time and space to find their own life before it ended. After they were on their own for a while, they told me what a rewarding experience it was to rediscover themselves. Selma, my 67-year-old client who had the courage to divorce after 40-plus years of a difficult marriage, told me, "I needed to create peace in my life and now I finally have it. I thought I couldn't do anything right. He was so critical of me. Now I've learned that I'm not as stupid as he thought I was!"

Contrary to popular belief, many women who need to end their marriages do quite well. Christiane Northrup, M.D., in talking about the end of her 25-year marriage said, "It's a paradox that my divorce was a personal tragedy and the best thing that ever happened to me." Renee, 57, told me, "I just went through the breakup of a 15-year marriage and I'm getting myself back. I'm getting rid of old baggage, whipping myself into shape again, and doing many of the things I enjoy that I had let slip away."

After careful consideration, and couples counseling, if you decide to divorce, take the following steps even before you see an attorney or mediator:

The Next Fifty Years

- Start saving money to pay for a lawyer.
- Open bank accounts in your own name.
- Establish your own credit.
- Keep a record of personal expenses.
- Gather as much information as possible about you and your spouse's financial situation.

More recently, divorce for women has come to seem tantamount to liberation, escape from enslavement to men and to their own misguided romanticism. Wendy Swallow said in her book, *Breaking Apart: A Memoir of Divorce,* "Now, I'm on my own. By standing alone in the world I stand more honestly, more nakedly, than ever before. It's my story now. I'm no longer a footnote in someone else's book."

If you were drawn to read this essay I assume you are divorcing, or thinking about it. Consider that your spouse may find this journal and it may not be a good idea to write your thoughts here. However, if you feel it's safe to do so, I've provided space below:

_____

_____

_____

_____

Trusting Yourself in Relationship

"Midlife is a time to recognize the pilgrim in us, that part of us which stumbles in confusion and wanders in the gray mist of unknowing. It is a time to grow in trust, believing that the stars that shine in our soul will lead and guide us to the future."

—Joyce Rupp, *Dear Heart, Come Home: The Path of Midlife Spirituality*

Each year, millions of older women seek new romantic connections after a divorce, widowhood, or the breakup of a long-term relationship. When contemplating a new relationship, many of us toss obstacles in our own paths. The biggest one is fear of putting trust in another partner. We don't trust our decision-making abilities. After divorce, for instance, some people remember only hurt, anger, and mistrust and forget the good times. The thought of finding a new partner rekindles memories of pain, rejection, and the loss of personal identity. Perhaps you've asked yourself, "Why take the risk? Why let love ruin my life again?" This line of questioning sets oneself up as a victim, one who's afraid to take a chance again.

Some women become less dependent on the men in their lives as they age (or evolve). Others become more dependent. To women, men sometimes seem like a different species. In general, women seem more afraid of being abandoned, as opposed to men, who are generally more afraid of being sucked into a merged oneness.

Other women find they become someone they don't recognize in their relationships with men. They resort to behaviors that validate their men at their own expense. Does your deep desire for love and acceptance make you unwilling or unable to share those parts of yourself you fear may seem too needy or difficult? Unfortunately, women learn that to preserve their relationships, they must keep more and more of their reactions to themselves and take a path away from authenticity, mutuality, and the truth of their experience.

Sex, of course, is a minefield today. Women are concerned to start a new relationship and they expect prospective sex partners to be tested for sexually transmitted diseases. One positive effect of this issue is a reluctance to indulge in the instant sex that hardly ever leads to a lasting relationship.

Maybe you believe you have little to offer in a new relationship. Janet told me she has a fear of being rejected: "I'm too old, so nobody will want me." Truth is, being older is now more of a plus than a minus. There are more people over age 50 today than at any other time in history. The world is full of people your age who are looking for a person like you.

Mature love is a stage in life when you choose someone not because he looks like a young Greek god, but because he stirs something in your heart. You are at a stage when you've become too sophisticated to fall for illusions. Gloria Steinem once said, "For me . . . aging has also brought freedom from romance; freedom from the ways in which your hormones distort your judgment."

How do you feel about this?

_____

_____

_____

_____

In what ways can you learn to trust yourself in a love relationship?

_____

_____

_____

_____

Dating after 50

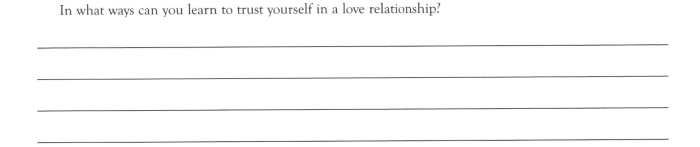

"If all you see are frogs, maybe you need new glasses."

–Rachelle Zuckerman, Ph.D., *Young at Heart: The Mature Woman's Guide to Finding and Keeping Romance*

What are the rules for dating after 50? I hate imposing rules. Aren't we too evolved and mature to be locked into rules? If there's any one rule to adhere to it's this: Be yourself and maintain an active interest in the world around you. Older women struggle with redefining themselves because the last time they were single was probably in their twenties. This hardly serves as a point of reference for single life after age 50.

How does dating after 50 differ from younger years? Well, for starters, we have access to the Internet, which is a great way to sort through hundreds of interesting men.

The Internet is one of the best matchmakers ever for women over 50. This rapidly expanding way to meet a date or mate is easy, inexpensive, and respectable, as well as fun. It saves time, too. Browse one or more of the many online dating services and check them out. Some of them offer one-week trial memberships for free.

One of my clients, a lovely, interesting woman of 61, began dating online about a year ago. During that first year she received over 300 responses to her ad. After carefully following safety guidelines, she went on dates with 23 of the most promising prospects, and is now engaged to a great guy.

With Internet dating, you need to follow some basic rules. Stay anonymous for as long as you feel okay doing so, regardless of his questions. Be less concerned for his feelings than for your own safety. The beauty of this technology is that you can hit the delete key if someone becomes inappropriate or invasive. If he refuses to give you his work and home numbers—if he won't say what he does (or did) for a living but insists on knowing where you live or work—end the conversation. Does hitting the delete key seem rude to you? Don't worry about it. With online dating, this is totally acceptable.

If you decide to meet him, use common sense and choose a crowded public place. Keep the meeting short, about one hour for the first date. Take yourself to and from the meeting place on your own. After taking a few smart precautions, you may even find come-hithers through an Internet dating service preferable to meeting strangers in smoky bars. Remember, relationships today need as much in-person time as they ever did to mature into real intimacy.

If you are wondering who would ever ask you out, you are clearly suffering from low self-esteem. Anyone can be desirable—first you need to believe you are. The mature men I interviewed for this book said in general the woman they find most attractive is the woman who knows who she is, who has a sense of playfulness and vitality. Women who do not neglect their health were also mentioned. If you have chronic health issues or a disability, are you less attractive? They told me not necessarily—it's the woman's attitude that's important.

One of my good friends says that when you're over 50 you should date much taller men—men you can look up to so your chins won't be as noticeable! Chins aside, it makes sense that you might be fearful of putting yourself out there in the "marketplace" after coming through a divorce or the death of a spouse. According to Mel and Pat Krantzler in *Learning to Love Again*, learning to love again progresses through an initial stage when just thinking about a new love relationship can feel too vulnerable an activity to the open wound in the heart. The signal you send to potential lovers is, "Don't come close to me. I've been hurt too much." Conversely, this stage may bring on a wild rush to marry an improved version or a clone of your former spouse in an effort to make yourself feel whole again. It's important to remember that a healthy relationship is not based on being part of another person, that each of us is already a whole person.

After a period of time, one recognizes that being a single person offers one opportunities to respond to new challenges in unexplored ways. Remembered pain from the former relationship begins to diminish in intensity. The realization emerges that you are now completely free to try new relationships. Eventually, the belief that you are only half a person declines. You are now a competent single individual. However, if you've lost a love relationship through death or divorce, the fear may persist that a close commitment will

The Next Fifty Years

end in disaster. Take heart—the courage to embrace an intimate relationship will eventually overpower your fear of its possible failure or loss.

As you begin to trust yourself more, you will ultimately begin to trust in others. As we grow older, every day becomes more precious. If you are alone and want to share your life with a special someone, open your heart cautiously, smile, explore with the intent to learn—enjoy and embrace life.

How do you feel about this?

_____

_____

_____

_____

What attributes do you bring to the dating table?

_____

_____

_____

_____

Choosing Commitment after 50

"The second time around has been not so much about correcting past mistakes as about the willingness to make new ones."

—Ana Veciana-Suarez

Many older women late in life are choosing to get married or live together in committed relationships. These relationships are described by observers and the couples themselves as peaceful, gratifying, liberating, and rich in companionship. These women typically are free from the pressures of working and raising families, and due to their added years of life experience, they are often highly aware of what they're looking for in a mate.

Life isn't all roses, however. Difficulties may come up because the adult children are concerned that a new spouse will usurp their role in decisions regarding care should their parent become sick, or that they may lose their inheritance. Despite the potential stumbling blocks, many people in late-life marriages say they have never been happier.

When lovers in their seventies and eighties marry, they do so quickly. To them, life is transient and more precious. Those who don't remarry usually find long-term relationships. Attachment is the sense of calm, peace, and security that you have with a long-term partner after the exciting but exhausting state of infatuation.

If you've had a marriage that was fulfilling, you might be more inclined to want to be married again, and you have a choice. Living together might be a good idea if you have considerations (practical and emotional) of Social Security, medical insurance, independence, and inheritance.

More than 200,000 women over 50 are headed for the altar; for most of them, it is the second time around. For some of them, it's actually the first time. A friend recently told me the story of a 51-year-old family member who married for the first time because it took her that long to find the right guy. We're even coming up with new definitions to describe these late-life marriages. The *Dictionary of the Future* by Faith Popcorn gives this definition: "Elderweds: People age 60 or older who are marrying for the first time or remarrying."

When we marry or live in a committed relationship after 50, we might not have 30 or 40 years to work out the kinks, so it's best to know each other well beforehand.

Also, it's important to consult with a financial advisor and/or an attorney. Serious relationships in later life are a bit more complicated financially than for younger couples. There may be family members to care for, such as children of a prior marriage, ex-spouses, parents. The couple may have heavy financial obligations, alimony payments, child support. They may have piled up assets in which others have a stake. Financial advisors say you might consider a prenuptial agreement if either one of you owns a business or has children. Then plan to change your will after getting married so you can update beneficiary designations on retirement plans and insurance policies.

Marriage and commitment at any age aren't easy. Creating a successful marriage can be the most difficult challenge of an adult's life. I think it's worth the effort. According to researchers, few accomplishments are more important to happiness, health, fulfillment, and satisfaction in life than a healthy marriage. On the other hand, few experiences in life are more defeating than an unsuccessful one.

The Next Fifty Years

If you think you're too old to have and maintain a love relationship, think again. My 70-plus friend Alma Garville, recently married, opened a fortune cookie while out to dinner on her honeymoon that said, "If you think you're too old to do something, do it anyway."

How do you feel about this?

_____

_____

_____

_____

If you had the opportunity to make a new commitment to either marriage or living together, would you?

_____

_____

_____

_____

7

Our Spiritual Self

"Lift us now on strong wings; encourage us to create more spaces where we can sit down together and weep and still be counted warriors."

—From a prayer by Ruth Cowan

In my practice I've seen women express a deep, previously unspoken desperation to connect with the spiritual self. They find there is a void in their lives and that aging is a much more challenging experience because of this void. The spiritual self of the aging woman is not necessarily nurtured in our religious institutions, although it can be. Community with others is essential for some, and for others this search has more to do with a private connection to the universe or an internal divinity.

I didn't use to think as much about my spiritual life as I do now. For many years I was too busy making a living, raising a family, and having all the anxieties that go along with those earlier years in a woman's life. Now my spiritual attitude colors everything I do, everything I think, everything I read. Adulthood is a time of continuing development and growth. In midlife, we come to a fork in the road of our lives. The values and goals that have served us well in the first half of our lives become increasingly irrelevant as family, career, and health considerations shift and change. Midlife is the time to give birth to a new way of being in the world.

As women in this country enjoy longer lives and better health than previous generations, and as the population inches toward being more senior than junior, we are becoming as interested in the effects of aging on the human spirit as on the human body.

Successful aging cannot be measured by the degree of one's retained youthfulness. The media would have you believe that an unlined face, a trim body, and a spring in your step are the yardsticks of achievement in old age, but those who look a little deeper know better. Embracing and discovering our spiritual self is a process of expanding consciousness and developing wisdom that can enable the older woman to become a radiant, vitally alive, and socially responsible elder.

The spiritual journey is a lifelong process of discovery. One of our most important tasks as maturing women is to find what spiritual truths and principles work best for us and which ones we intend to live out our lives with. The outcome of this endeavor is not necessarily to find which religion you should join, or which faith you should switch to.

Whether we reach up for God, look out into the world for the goddess, or seek a divine spark within, we need to honor and value our personal search, understanding that the attributes of aging facilitate and enhance the search. We each look at the world in different ways, colored by our respective life experiences. Through a lens of perception that views and reflects back the world in a unique way for each of us, we consider the role of spirituality in our lives with varying degrees of intensity and involvement. At each phase of our continuing evolution, some spiritual truths will work better for us than others. We have differing concepts of faith, and each of us must come to our own meaningful conclusion.

But I think we all agree on one thing—as we age, our spirituality grows and becomes increasingly relevant to the imminence of death, which creates a deeper appreciation of life.

Our spiritual self is an essential aspect of ourselves—you may call it the higher self, real self, the center, or the God within. It feels like "home" when we connect with it. Psychoanalyst Carl Jung used the simple word "Self" to indicate that this place within us is connected to that which is greater than our individual and conscious identity.

When you connect to your Self, you can face whatever is associated with aging with added strength and humor. Your belief in yourself and your value has grown with time. Your life is joined to others and to something greater than your self. Your life ends up having a more compelling personal grace and naturalness that is unaffected by your passing years.

Hopefully, the topics in this section will help guide you in focusing and thinking about some attitudes and activities whose by-product is joy as we proceed along the path of aging. The topics covered include seeing yourself as a goddess, living an authentic life, discovering your hidden strengths, liberating yourself from the material, the role of religion in longevity, slowing your pace and quieting your life in order to promote soul growth, and the spiritual issues that come up for all of us around death and dying.

Spirituality and Health

"Knowing and praising God makes the 50-plus woman delightfully different. . . Praise lifts our face and . . . our spirit."

—Shirley Mitchell, *Fabulous after 50: Finding Fulfillment for Tomorrow*

A study once confirmed that people who go to church, synagogue, or mosque regularly tend to have lower blood pressure, stronger immune systems, and lower rates of cancer, heart disease, and mental illness—they live longer as a result. The study examined a wide range of social, economic, and lifestyle factors to find out which ones contributed to living longer. What stood out as a major factor was frequent attendance at religious services. The researchers found that the life expectancy gap between those who attend more than once a week and those who never attend is over seven years.

Such people are more energetic and less likely to feel depressed or anxious. Some studies have shown spiritual beliefs to be more important for good health than not smoking. That's a striking finding. People who pray or meditate experience the relaxation response—a drop in blood pressure, heart rate, and levels of stress hormones such as cortisol. Prayer and meditation also cause an increase in alpha and theta waves. These electrical impulses in the brain are associated with relaxation. Even if you do not pray or meditate, having religious or spiritual beliefs can reduce anxiety.

One theory is that the social support from spiritual communities such as churches, meditation groups, or yoga classes helps people buffer the harmful effects of stress. Not all spiritual beliefs are equally beneficial. People with positive spiritual beliefs, such as the idea that God represents love and forgiveness, do better than those who believe in harsh divine punishment.

While factors that often accompany religious activity, such as strong social ties and healthier lifestyles, play a role in lengthening life, the researchers say there is something more going on. Perhaps what's going on is hinted at in the Bible (Isa. 46:4): "Even to your old age, I shall be the same, and even to your graying years I shall bear you! I have done it, and I shall carry you; And I shall bear you, and I shall deliver you."

Suppose attending a religious service just isn't for you. You can increase your spirituality and get some great benefit by setting aside 20 minutes daily for quiet time. Spend the time meditating, listening to music, or simply allow-

The Next Fifty Years

ing yourself to think about the wonders of nature, a memorable line from a poem, etc. Read spiritual books, poetry, or essays. Read the works of philosophers or theologians. Be part of a small spiritual community that gives to others. Nearly all of the world's religions and spiritual traditions emphasize charitable giving. When you share with others, you form deeper connections with a world that is greater than yourself.

How do you feel about this?

_____

_____

_____

_____

Is it time to take your spiritual growth more seriously? Would it help to attend a regular religious service or to do something else?

_____

_____

_____

Spirit in the Silence

"I know the gifts of Spirit not only when I hear the rippling of tongues but also in the gift of silence, when understanding and joy come without words."

—Madeleine L'Engle, *The Irrational Season*

As I write this, I'm at a friend's picturesque beach house on Plum Island, Massachusetts, where the silence is palpable. I don't often realize how much I miss the silence until I'm immersed in it as I am this morning. The sun is a bright globe peeking over the horizon and I hear the tranquilizing hymn of the waves lulling the shoreline. I feel the reverence of the pulsing sunrise, the litany of the ocean's expanse, the laughing liturgy of seagulls, the ocean mist baptizing my face. Age does not matter in these sacramental moments of connection with spirit.

In the silence I feel my own life's pulse. I wait. I listen. I understand that I am in a spiritual realm that I did not create. I understand that I am luxuriously immersed in my choice to be in solitude and to be in the fullness of my own presence. I do silence well and I am proud of my accomplishment.

I promise my maturing self that this will be a priceless gift I give to me each day. Each day I will carve out of chaos a silence where I listen for spirit to rise in me, noiseless as sunrise on Plum Island.

"If we never pause long enough to get to know the silence, how will we know the possibilities it contains?"

—Sue Bender, *Stretching Lessons*

Journal below about your experience with spirit in the silence:

_____

_____

_____

_____

_____

_____

_____

Obituaries and Inspiration

"Fall was coming. . . . Sadie still held her vigil in the window, but now a shawl was curled about her shoulders to ward off the chill."

—Sarah L. Delany, *On My Own at 107*

Lately, I find my self turning to the *New York Times* obituaries to find inspiration in the lives of interesting, creative, vital older women who have lived long into their lives. Here are some of my favorites:

Sophie—96, a leading Orthodox Christian educator whose life encompassed the history of twentieth-century Russia and the experience of Russian émigrés, died in Valley Cottage, New York, on Friday. Author of many books, at 77 Sophie wrote her memoir *Many Worlds: A Russian Life*. At the time of her death she was working as president of Religious Books for Russia, and she continued traveling and lecturing into her nineties. The obituary is full of her life's accomplishments, and what impressed me most is that she kept on keeping on and getting on with it.

Evelyn—90. "Beloved wife . . . Loving mother and grandmother . . . Former Executive Secretary . . . As a Gray Lady during WWII she comforted the troops when they returned from battle. . . ." Beloved wife (and widow). Loving mother (someone's daughter) and grandmother. Executive secretary (the great woman behind the man), and Gray Lady (a rainbow full of color, a gift to the traumatized). So much more we don't know about her 90 years of life. This makes me want to call her family and friends and say, "Tell me more, tell me more."

Sylvia—89. "Beloved wife of the late Samuel, formerly of New York City. Loving mother of Eleanor and Bill. Dear sister of Mildred and Leon. Loving grandmother of Deborah, Will, Sarah, and Rebecca. Caring great aunt of Jeff . . ." Beloved wife (and widow). Loving mother (someone's daughter). Loving grandmother. Caring great aunt. Tell me more. Tell me more.

Lorraine—97. "Died peacefully at home in the arms of her beloved husband of 53 wonderful years . . . Loving mother . . . adored niece . . . devoted friend to many. Lorraine, an effervescent woman of great charm, intelligence, courage, spirit, understanding, compassion, wit, and humor, had the marvelous gift to make people laugh and feel alive. Lorraine will be deeply missed by all."

I wonder how my obituary will read? Will I be remembered as beloved, loving, and caring of someone? As one "whose life encompassed"—what? Maybe I'll write my own obituary, store it with my will with strict instructions to use it word for word. "She lived, she died, and in-between she tried to make a difference in the world." No. Maybe I shouldn't be selfish. Let them (whoever's left) write it up. It will probably help them grieve. Hopefully they knew who I was. Hopefully, I knew who I was.

Unless you're totally unselfconscious, you hit a stage about age 50 when you start to realize that you're not going to be here forever. Our process of aging of course is taking us toward our own deaths. The older you are, the more this becomes a daily awareness. Or a daily avoidance. Mary C. Morrison says in one of her books, "The concept of death can set us free—free to live fully in our time, free to be human beings again at last, aware of our end and of the measure of our days."

The message that no matter what you do, you'll die anyway is neither depressing nor hopeless. It's a challenge, an invitation to come back to something more meaningful than an impossible attempt to recapture youth. Accepting the inevitability and reality of death makes it possible to really live, to get our priorities straight.

How do you feel about this?

_____

_____

_____

_____

What would you like your obituary to say about you?

_____

_____

_____

_____

_____

Journaling the Days

"Another reason for writing in your diary is to discover that the ideas in you are an inexhaustible fountain."

—Brenda Ueland, *If You Want to Write*

Annie Dillard once said, "How we spend our days is how we spend our lives." Inspired by this quote, I've decided to be more intentional in my journaling, to explore just how I'm spending my days. Like currency, am I spending too much on the minutia or the irrelevant? Am I spending well past my limit? Creating too much debt and not reimbursing myself?

Journaling is a way to keep track of how we spend our days. Something like a spiritual balance sheet. Tuesday I spent too much time in contemplation and not enough time getting the work done. On Thursday I spent too much time getting the mundane done and not enough time in reflection. Journaling has taught me the fine art of balance, and the discipline has helped me become more aware of who I am.

Every so often I hear someone say, "I just don't know where today went!" A lament that brings me up short. A reminder that the days are numbered—just so many left in the account. Consider keeping two journals—one for everyday contemplation and reporting; another entitled "Things I Love," starting each line or paragraph with the words, "I love . . ." My first entry says, "I love writing with a fountain pen." My second entry says, "I love the way my adult son kisses me on the forehead." Another says, "I love the first buds of spring on the maple trees that enclose my yard." Glue in pictures from magazines, or photos you love. A journal will help you explore who you are by identifying what you love, and how you spend your days.

How do you feel about this?

_____

_____

How are you spending your days and what do you love?

_____

_____

_____

_____

_____

_____

_____

Intuition and Wisdom

"There are things I know, things I have learned from deep inside, from other women; from holding children; from looking into the eyes of dying patients and tending their bodies when life has departed; from living my life listening to the voice in the river or the wind, the caw of a crow, the stillness of deep night."

—Janet F. Quinn, *I Am a Woman Finding My Voice*

In general, the educational institutions that teach us how to use our minds, and the organizations in which we use them, have not been structured to nurture intuition. To move successfully through the first years of adulthood, many women were encouraged (or forced) to view the world as a rational, competitive, hierarchical, patriarchal, and materialistic place. Fortunately, now that you're in the second half of your life, you're ready to abandon that limiting view of the world. Now you're ready to ask deeper questions, and to learn to listen to your inner voice. I believe with all my heart that a woman's innate intuition sharpens and wisdom deepens as we become older.

If you listen carefully, your inner wisdom will guide you in ways to care for your aging body, your mind, and your spirit. No more discounting what you know is true about your world and yourself! When you feel an intuitive pull to call a friend or relative, follow through. When you feel a certain decision isn't for your highest good, change your mind. If you're asked to do something or go somewhere that doesn't feel right in your gut, refuse to do it.

Now is the time to fully own your intuitive wisdom and power.

How do you feel about this?

_____

_____

_____

_____

Write about an intuition you had about a situation that came true:

_____

_____

_____

_____

_____

_____

_____

_____

Finding Peace

"What, then, is 'spirituality,' defined not in the usual way but as it pertains to the woman wanting to find peace with the universe? It is a feeling that the world is basically beautiful and filled with wonder, that there is a dimension of life beyond what is known."

—Mary McConnell, *Still Dancing: Life Choices and Challenges for Women*

At 65, Selma's life goal was to experience something she had rarely known—peace, plain and simple. She had endured for 45 years an emotionally abusive marriage and it needed to end if she was ever going to experience peace. I thought to myself, what a simple request of the universe—wanting to live a peaceful life; yet how for many women, it remains an elusive state of being. When Selma finally separated from her husband and subsequently acquired a small condo of her own, the first thing she reported feeling when she walked into her new living space was peace.

I don't think we necessarily need to make as drastic a life change as divorce to find peace. Yet finding peace does require a change of attitude and a willingness to be proactive in the search for it.

Jane, 57, is the mother of two teenagers. She's seeking peace also—the kind of peace that comes with solitude and time for herself. Her tonic is the arts. She finds a peace there that is helping her navigate the stresses of motherhood and aging. "It's hard to stay in an unsettled place when gazing at a magnificent painting or listening to music I love," she told me. "Even taking a half hour or so to fool around with paints or play the piano diverts my attention to a more centered place."

If we are mothers, the reality is that we may have to put off finding great chunks of peace and solitude until the children are grown and gone. For Lynne Zielinski (author of *Chocolate for a Woman's Spirit*) peace comes in the form of the little things. She writes, "I am so grateful for the gifts of my autumn—opportunities to experience simple pleasures that, in times past, scurried by unnoticed in the maelstrom of raising children."

For me, being close to nature makes me realize that no matter how I feel, the Sun still rises and sets each day. It's taken some discipline, but sitting on a bench in my garden, strolling on a beach, or lying on a hillside and gazing at the sky gives me a sense of peace and a connection to something greater than myself. As I age I am more and more apt to turn off the radio and TV and to bask in the silence. I also feel more peaceful in an uncluttered, organized living space.

How do you feel about this?

_____

_____

_____

_____

In what ways can you create some peace in your life?

_____

_____

_____

_____

Choosing to Be Authentic

"The choices we make determine who we become, offering us the possibility of leading an authentic life."

—Jean Shinoda Bolen, *Crossing to Avalon*

My most memorable and life-filling moments were connected to my years performing in the theater. However, life brought me financial responsibility and demands that caused me to work too many unfulfilling years as an office manager and associate in a consulting company. As we mature, we come to realize that for much of our lives, work has formed the structure of our time, and most of our activities have been organized from outside ourselves rather than from within. As a younger woman I conformed to society's expectations and yearned for approval. Now I'm free to feel good about who I am and what I do.

Some of the many gifts of the midlife passage include the death of our attempts to control and letting go of protective masks, letting go of manipulative behaviors, toxic relationships, unrealistic self-images, unhealthy addictions, protective illusions, old gods, and expectations. As older women we can choose to be authentic in all we do.

Anne Morrow Lindbergh wrote in *Gift from the Sea,* "Perhaps middle age is, or should be, a period of shedding shells: the shell of ambition, the shell of material accumulations and possessions, the shell of the ego." Often we hide out in comfy, unchallenging jobs that surround us with pleasant people, provide a paycheck, and seem benign enough, except that we're not expressing our authentic selves one tiny bit.

Why do we keep something about ourselves a secret? What we have difficulty acknowledging is usually the very thing we need to confront and resolve. When we deny parts of ourselves, we are limiting the options we have in life. There is an insidious link between hiding and self-sabotage.

The great irony about hiding is that we think it will simplify our lives. However, hiding takes tremendous energy you could be spending in other more fulfilling areas of your life. Stop putting up with situations you hate and stop making excuses to yourself and anyone else who'll listen, while ignoring the persistent need for authenticity.

My friend Alex remembers her mother as a woman "who never got to express herself and felt threatened because I was so expressive." Her mother and my mother were part of a generation of women in the 1950s and 1960s who dedicated their lives to their kids and never got to find out who they were as creative beings. Consequently, a lot of us as children got shushed and learned to associate full self-expression with shame and "inappropriate" behavior.

Fortunately, when you finally let yourself be authentic, the sky does not fall. I know from embracing my own authenticity that there is a queasiness at first, followed by a lightness and a sense that you are in the right place. Things begin to unfold and miracles happen.

You may wonder, "Who will love me if they know who I really am?" For those of us who like to hide, that is the question. The answer is, not everyone and possibly everyone. The deeper you dig within yourself and the more you expose, the more you connect with the rest of the world. You end up finding out a shocking and beautiful truth: There are people out there who really do want to hear what you have to say and who love you even more because you are fully who you were meant to be.

How do you feel about this?

_____

_____

_____

_____

What are you hiding about yourself?

_____

_____

_____

_____

If you expressed your authentic self, what would happen to your life?

_____

_____

_____

_____

Are You a Goddess?

"Social-wise, you can go ethnic anywhere,
in a sari or a muumuu or a caftan,
if it's more comfortable, and who cares if
you look like a refugee from the sixties."

—Peg Bracken, *On Getting Old for the First Time*

My sister, Marilyn, and I began to play with the idea that all women are goddesses after age 50—that is, we are powerful and beautiful and come in all different sizes and shapes. Just in case you're interested in discerning whether or not you qualify as a goddess, we put together the following lists (with room to add ideas of your own).

Goddesses wear (if they want to):

- beautiful, silky caftans
- earrings that swing and make soft tinkling sounds
- sequins in the daytime
- long skirts with slits
- colored eye shadow
- comfortable, supportive, attractive shoes that don't hurt
- clothes that feel creamy, soft, and nurturing
- velour, chenille, fleece, and velvet whenever they want to
- beautiful bras and sexy panties to bed under their sleepwear (especially if they are sharing their bed with a lover)
- whatever colors make them feel good, happy, and alive
- more than one ring on each hand

Goddesses never wear:

- tight waistbands or tight anything
- what the designers tell them to
- high, spiky heels
- spandex
- double-knit polyester anything
- days of the week underwear
- big hair
- cinch belts
- ponytails (braids, yes)

Goddesses can have:

- 15 flavors of tea in the house
- chocolate anywhere, anytime
- lip gloss in the pocket of every coat and jacket
- wind chimes hanging anywhere they want

The Next Fifty Years

- Christmas lights up all year long in the bedroom, kitchen, or living room
- McDonald's Happy Meals for lunch (or buy them just for the toys)
- Pepsi and ginger snaps for breakfast
- picnics in bed
- as many lovers as they want
- a good laugh whenever they want (even if they're alone and watching Three Stooges marathons on TV)
- 25-watt bulbs in every lamp in the house (and dust less when company is coming)
- 150-watt bulbs for reading erotic poetry and *Playgirl* magazine
- as many candles, incense, and bags of potpourri as they can afford

---

Goddesses must:

- be outrageous
- have their own computer
- get a facial once a year and a pedicure at least twice a year
- have a contingency plan for running away from home if necessary
- remember that round is a shape
- flirt all they want, especially with younger men

In Christina Biaggi's *In the Footsteps of the Goddess*, Susan Menje, a Wiccan high priestess and artist, said, "We are all the Goddess in many forms and many guises." Here's a final thought from Marianne Williamson in *A Woman's Worth*: "What mature women want is this: the lightheartedness of our youth with the added depth our suffering of the past few years has given us. Through the grace of the Goddess, it is within our grasp to have both." I for one believe her.

How do you feel about this?

In what ways can you embrace your "Goddess-self"?

_____

_____

_____

_____

Liberation from Material Things

"The fewer things you own, the more time you have for the important stuff. I want to go through life with only three of everything—one to wear and one to wash and a spare (except for panty liners). I want to own only what I need."

—Alma Garville, 76

Besides her quote above, my friend Alma asked me, "Why do we need so many towels, nightgowns, and bedsheets? Why so many groceries when the stores are open 24-7? Why stock up?" She made me think.

Sometimes it feels as if my possessions own me instead of me owning them. They call to me: Wash me, dust me, polish me, pack me away for the winter, move me, wear me, listen to me! How can we get to any kind of spiritual illumination or growth when we're so darn busy taking care of houses, attics, basements, and storage bins full of the detritus of the first 50 years of our lives?

An 80-year-old rabbi I once studied with came into class one day and announced, "I have given away all the books in my library." I was stunned. What is a rabbi (or any religious professional for that matter) without a library? When we asked why, he replied, "Because the books were all talking to me at the same time!" I think of him every time I look around my house.

A lot of my older female friends and clients feel that if a large enough number of people go through a shift from the material to a more psychological and spiritual point of view, then the culture will move along this path. There's no doubting that either spirituality is a fad right now or something significant and profound is happening. I think probably a little bit of both is going on.

How do you feel about this?

_____

_____

_____

_____

Make a list of some of the material things you'd like to be free from:

_____

_____

_____

_____

_____

_____

_____

_____

8

Our Creative Self

"The most insidious and common manifestation of repressed creativity in women is depression."

—C. Diane Ealy, *The Women's Book of Creativity*

Without a doubt, if you shift attention to your creative source, it will create a powerful healing effect on your physiology, spirituality, and ultimately your psychology. Creative activity can even help us climb out of the pit of depression.

Creative women are especially at risk of depression because they have often had their dreams and ideas discounted by peers and teachers at an early age. Despite this, a growing number of older women are delving for the first time into artistic expression, and their creativity is changing. They find that being creative is very invigorating and challenging. As a result, they discover their uniqueness and begin to get a much larger vision of what gives meaning and value to their lives.

The older woman is more than just a physical body, a brain, or a social unit; she also carries within her a remarkable, authentic, hidden self that can contribute greatly to the creative process. Dancer/choreographer Martha Graham said it best: "There is a vitality, a life force, a quickening that is translated through you into action, and because there is only one of you in all time, this expression is unique."

Research shows that creativity has a direct impact on health and longevity. An issue of *Mind/Body Health Newsletter* in 1999 said that studies had been done on the effect that writing had on chronic illnesses such as asthma and arthritis. In patients with rheumatoid arthritis who wrote about stressful life experiences, writing significantly reduced the severity of their arthritis. The article said that patients in the experimental group had less joint pain, swelling, and tenderness, and were better able to carry out their normal, everyday activities.

Until recently, creativity was viewed as the domain of only a privileged few—those blessed with talents that most mortals lack. If you were an artist in your younger years, it was assumed that once you turned 50, the decline in creativity was accelerated and remorseless. Today, a new understanding about creativity is emerging. Current research shows it as something that can be nurtured in virtually everyone, regardless of age.

For a variety of reasons, many women don't discover their potential until they grow older. One reason is that many women are too busy working and raising families to seriously pursue creative arts. Someone once said that "retirement is like a patron of the arts." Time, which has been viewed as the enemy of the old, is actually more plentiful in later life. Rather than old age being a time of constriction, it can be a time of serious expansion and liberation.

For some of us, it can take the accumulated wisdom of a lifetime to have something to say artistically. Aging can bring confidence and courage. Older artists are often willing to take greater risks than younger ones. A young woman of 21 might say, "I'm not going to do that. I'll look like an idiot for trying." Whereas a 65-year-old woman might say, "I'm going to give that a try—what've I got to lose?"

When you make art as an older woman, you're immersing yourself in history, memory, stories, and relationships. This is an opportunity to place yourself in your own life. You don't necessarily need to have training—you simply need to be open to revelation.

Even in the face of illness, creativity can be a response to digging down into the spirit to try to transcend pain. Just as too much sustained stress is harmful to your health, sustained attention to something you really love and find fulfilling has the converse effect.

Among other creative pursuits, this section encourages the reader to think about writing a book, a poem, a journal. It reminds the reader that creativity can take many forms in everyday life, and encourages her to consider how her attitude towards creativity can be self-defeating and that it's never too late in one's life to create.

It's Never Too Late to Create!

"As you get older, you want to pull things together—put all the fragments into something like a novel."

—Harriet Doerr

How many times have you said to yourself, "I wish I had . . ." or "I wish I could . . ." Well, is it too late? If blind painters can paint, if the hearing-impaired can write and perform music, if the crippled can choreograph a dance, what's to keep you from being creative? Your age? Stop complaining and start creating!

At the age of 104, retired teacher Sarah Delany collaborated with her sister Dr. Bessie Delany (then 102) to write the *New York Times* best-seller *Having Our Say: The Delany Sisters' First 100 Years*. Their book became a Broadway hit, and at 105 and 103 years of age, they published a sequel! You think *you're* too old? Pooh.

Haven't we been through a lot so far? We can create our best out of seeing the world through our individual and unique lifelong experiences. We've seen so much more of the world at our age that we bring even more juice, wisdom, and fire to whatever it is we create at this time in our lives.

Here are some inspirational women artists for you to think about:

- Grandma Moses was still busy painting at 100.
- Jessica Tandy won an Oscar at age 81.
- Imogen Cunningham, an accomplished American photographer, was still teaching at the Art Institute of San Francisco in her nineties.
- Hilda Doolittle, poet and writer, wrote *Helen in Egypt*, considered one of her strongest works, at the age of 75.

These women didn't allow themselves to fold up, sit in a chair, and wait for Meals on Wheels. Even if you're waiting for your meal to arrive, you can still create while you wait. Rebecca Latimer said in *You're Not Old until You're Ninety*: "As for expecting to live forever, I don't, and the way it takes me is to make me feel in a hurry to get done all I want to do while I'm still here."

How do you feel about this?

_____

_____

_____

_____

What creative project can you start today?

_____

_____

_____

_____

Claiming the Creative Self

"I'm a singer who wants to be a writer, and a writer who wants to grow up to be an artist. I don't want to do anything in the same way I did it before."

—Letty Cottin Pogrebin, *Getting Over Getting Older: An Intimate Journey*

An article appeared in the Arts section of the *New York Times* a while ago about Joni Mitchell, one of my favorite singers who became an artist (she's in her 60s now). In a report card note, her sixth grade teacher wrote, "Joan should pay attention to other subjects than art." Half a century later, Joni Mitchell went back to her hometown and brought 500 of her paintings, drawings, and photographs with her. Eighty-seven pieces were chosen for a show in the public gallery there.

Her teacher's remarks touched on something in me long forgotten: how people, early in my life, affected my dreams and career decisions. When I mentioned my desire to be an actress at age 15, my parents said I'd be better off getting a "real job." Later in life, when I confessed that I wanted to be a writer, they reminded me how many of them were starving.

So, is it too late in your second 50 years to began reclaiming the artist within you? Think back to what was said to the artist in you—rail against the negative dictates—become militant. Get angry and go paint. Paint anger. Paint the face of the person who told you that you couldn't paint, then go sell the portrait in your hometown gallery!

Melody Beattie in *Journey to the Heart* writes, "Who told you you weren't creative? Stand tall, speak up, and tell them they're wrong. Own your creative powers. Allow your creativity to heal and flourish." I say, go to the karaoke bar and sing. Dance like Isadora Duncan in your bare feet, color outside the lines, and break the rules.

How do you feel about this?

_____

_____

_____

_____

How can you reclaim and express your creative self?

_____

_____

_____

Creativity and Health

"It's a terrible thing in women's culture that you're supposed to be dead after menopause. . . . Since I was 60 I've written more and had better energy and more energy than I ever had in my life."

—Meridel Le Sueur, poet

Expressing the natural, vibrant force that is our creativity can improve our health, both physically and mentally. Creativity boosts our mood and increases our morale. Creativity has a way of challenging the brain to relieve mood and sleep disorders. Creativity strengthens the connections between brain cells and assists our memory. It offers a fresh way to respond to problems and may allow us to transcend them. Having a creative life can make it easier to face adversity, such as the loss of a spouse and or serious illness. With a fresh perspective, our emotions become more resilient. Capitalizing on creativity promotes a positive sense of well-being that can boost the immune system helping us to fight disease.

Stuck energy equals poor health, especially stuck *creative* energy. A colleague of mine, now a singer in her twenties, once kept putting off her desire to sing and developed one health issue after another that showed up around the throat area. A client with cancer told me of her desire to create her own line of jewelry and when she did, her cancer went into remission. I suffered with headaches for years before I realized that the stuck energy in my head had to become a book.

During the second half of one's life, women who devoted their lives to their families, and some who worked outside the home, can revisit long-postponed interests. Only in our later years do most women gain the self-confidence to explore their own creativity. Let's face it, creativity requires an acceptance of your uniqueness and of being imperfect. With the wisdom that comes with maturity, we know ourselves better and we learn that making a mistake won't destroy our self-image or the opinions others have of us. So get creative and get healthy.

How do you feel about this?

_____

_____

_____

_____

Have you identified stuck energy in your creative life and what would you like to do about it?

_____

_____

_____

_____

_____

Dancing from a Wheelchair

"The work of artists teaches us so many things about the sustaining role of creativity throughout our lives. For many older artists, that playful, free spirit helps them to find solutions to the problems of their changing abilities."

—Alexandra Stoddard, *The Art of the Possible*

The simple definition of creativity is to bring into existence something new and valued—a symphony or life-changing invention. However, what you bring into existence can also be a recipe, a well-planned vegetable garden, or a time-saving new route to a friend's house. Gene Cohen, M.D., author of *The Creative Age: Awakening Human Potential in the Second Half of Life*, said, "As the lead researcher of a 25-year study on creativity . . . in more than 200 senior citizens, I learned that anyone can be creative." Despite those findings, some of us think we're too old and we put obstacles in our way.

In a *New York Times* article (August 14, 2000) entitled "A Dance Icon Sees a Lovely Now in the Mirror," Jennifer Dunning tells us about Katherine Dunham, star of countless international dance tours and Broadway and Hollywood musicals from the 1940s on. Although 91 and wheelchair bound, Dunham leads a busy life teaching dance classes! She participates frequently in seminars and is at work on the next installment of her autobiography, to be called *The Minefield*. She will soon be involved in the renovation of her theater museum in East St. Louis, where she also maintains a school.

Maybe you feel crippled in other ways. Perhaps life is too busy for you to slow down enough to find your creative spirit. Susan K. Perry, Ph.D., author of *Writing in Flow: Keys to Enhanced Creativity*, talks about a 71-year-old woman who "knew she'd write her life story someday. But her real life kept getting in the way. She sold real estate and bred show horses, married four times and raised three daughters." Now that the children are grown and she's retired from real estate, she has started writing short stories and a memoir. She found she has a natural flair for clear writing and she's having a blast.

How do you feel about this?

_____

_____

_____

_____

What obstacles to your creativity are in your way?

_____

_____

_____

_____

Put It on Paper!

"Whatever coaxes us out of hiding, to write, record, and express, is a revolutionary act. It says that we believe our lives count."

—Sark, *Succulent Wild Woman*

Don't scare yourself. If you want to write a poem, *write* a poem. Write a journal, write an epic or a screenplay. Don't worry about who will see it. If someday you decide to share it, then share. Write whatever you write for yourself. Write for no particular reason or for a way to explore your feelings. Anne Morrow Lindbergh once wrote, "I began these pages for myself, in order to think out my own particular pattern of living, my own individual balance of life, work, and human relationships." Anais Nin wrote many journals from the time she was 63 to the time of her death at age 74. Her journals provide us with a candid, passionate account of her voyage of self-discovery.

Once you start putting it (whatever it is) on paper, of course you'll judge yourself. Please be kind to yourself. Even published writers have been known to judge themselves. Sue Bender, 66 and author of two of my favorite books, said in *Stretching Lessons*, "I've written two books using struggle as my method. But, after seventeen years of this single-minded obsession with writing, I still didn't think of myself as a writer."

Perhaps setting your mind on writing will give you motivation for life. Sarah Delany, 107, said, "I'm going to get to work on another book! . . . it's not ambition that drives me. It's having a sense of purpose. A reason to get up every morning."

Begin, and then begin again. Put it on paper, scrap paper and Bic ballpoint, unlined craft paper and magic markers, loose-leaf paper, fine linen writing paper and a fountain pen, paper napkins, small spiral notebooks with angels on the cover, newsprint, large journals, desk blotters, book margins with pencil. Discover yourself, embrace your soul, your unique talent. Put it on paper.

How do you feel about this?

_____

_____

_____

_____

Use these lines to put something on paper (e.g., an idea for a poem, a book, an essay)

_____

_____

_____

_____

_____

_____

_____

_____

_____

_____

_____

Creativity and Longevity

"To be creative, you must periodically recharge your inner resources of imagination. No matter how busy you are, you must set aside an hour or two every week to do something for yourself—something you enjoy. . . . Creativity is like a child within you."

—Julia Cameron, *The Artist's Way*

Blood pumps when we do something creative. Vessels open in the brain, circulation renews the spirit. What is creativity? If you are stuck thinking it's only smearing paint on canvas, writing a novel, or chipping a sculpture out of marble, then your creative spark might end up stuck forever. Isn't planting a garden an act of creativity? Writing a letter to a friend? Isn't setting the table with a pretty pattern or bright colors an act of creativity every bit as remarkable as oil paint on canvas? Isn't a beautifully made bed, an artfully arranged bookshelf, or a collection of candle holders artwork?

We live longer, happier lives if we take the time to be creative. We manifest health if we are willing to see the way we live as a creative expression. Even the small, tedious chores can be seen this way. Arranging the dishes in the dish drainer, folding the clothes, polishing your nails. Vacuum the carpet and notice the lines and swirls the vacuum makes. Dust the furniture but make a doodle in the dust before you wipe it away. Hang clothes to dry, watch as they flap about in the breeze against a blue sky.

Look around you. You don't even have to buy a box of crayons. Everywhere your eyes land there is a palette of color, myriad textures. I say, even if you view your world through a different lens every day, even if you see only the rainbows in the soap bubbles as you wash the frying pan—you are living a creative life—a life worth living for a long time.

How do you feel about this?

_____
_____
_____
_____

What can you do to live life more creatively?

_____
_____
_____
_____

Name one activity or object in your life that is a creative expression of who you are:

_____

Write a Poem

"Allowing poetry to create itself through me is a mystical experience that has given me joy all my life."

—Marilyn Houston, writer and poet

Perhaps you've never expressed yourself in poetry before. If you haven't, try it, you may really like it. Writing poetry can be fun and writing a simple poem that reflects your authentic, evolving self can do wonders to put life in perspective. Don't worry about grammar, spelling, or making sense. Try using the lines below to write a poem that expresses your thoughts and feelings about aging:

_____
_____
_____

_____

_____

_____

_____

_____

_____

_____

_____

Write a Book?

"Sometimes I believe these books are already written and my job is simply to allow them to come through me. My job is to get out of my own way."

—Sue Grafton, *Writing Mysteries: A Handbook*

How many times have you said to yourself, "If I only had the time I'd . . ." Fill in the blank. Maybe you filled in that blank with "I'd write a book," or "I'd write my memoirs," or "I'd keep a journal." So, what are you waiting for? Isn't it time to start if you haven't already? And if you've started a book, what's keeping you from finishing it? How many blank journals do you have that you've never written in because you think someone might find them when you're dead? So what?

Don't think you have the time? Julia Cameron, screenwriter and author of *The Artist's Way*, advises, "If you are interested in writing a book, write for a few minutes every day. Set aside a small amount of time and don't allow yourself to be distracted. After a few weeks you'll be encouraged by how much you have accomplished." Oh, and I love what Frances Weaver, author of *The Girls with the Grandmother Faces*, says, "Until we reached this wondrous age, we had not enough time of our own to sit down in a quiet place, collect our thoughts, let our imagination and memory float free, and enjoy our own heads. Now we can do that, and we write." Think you've got nothing relevant to say at your age? You're wrong. But why not write anyway? The act of writing will be its own reward.

Don't think you can get published? Then self-publish. Investigate an electronic publisher. Some will sell your work to Internet users in return for royalties of 50 percent. Self-publishers or cooperative publishers will design a cover, print and bind your book, assign an ISBN number, and tell you how to market it. An older woman I know writes poetry, prints out copies on her computer, staples them together, and gives them as gifts. These days there is just no excuse for not getting your work out there.

How do you feel about this?

_____

_____

_____

_____

What can you start writing about today?

_____

_____

_____

_____

What would the title of your book be?

_____

9

Our Health

"Our study . . . literally gave people something to live for. We need not fear that a long life automatically implies lifelong confinement in a nursing home."

—Thomas T. Perls and Margery Hutter Silver, *Living to 100*

Our tendency in this country is to treat old age like a problem desperately in need of a remedy. However, fewer Americans are becoming chronically disabled as they age. It's a trend, says AARP, "with powerfully positive implications for untold millions of aging Americans and for U.S. society as a whole." The odds of staying independent into old age and of staying out of a nursing home have been getting better with each passing year. What's behind the trend? Experts say there are a number of factors at work, among them: increasing education, improvements in maternal nutrition and public health, fewer people smoking, new drugs for heart disease and hypertension, healthier lifestyles, and advances in medical technology.

Obviously, getting old is mainly a matter of avoiding illness, and genes have a lot to do with that. But so does our behavior. According to researchers, making a big deal out of small troubles and slothful physical habits can reduce our genetic life expectancy by about ten years. Researchers are hoping that advances in biogenetics will reduce disability from genetically linked, progressive diseases such as Alzheimer's and Parkinson's.

Today's healthy 70-year-old women are doing what 50-year-olds did a generation ago. It's not necessarily about how we live but about how well we're able to live. More than half of baby boomers will live past 85, but we've got to exercise regularly and diet wisely. Maybe we can prevent some of the chronic illness we face along the way.

This section will explore health issues that affect the brain, our breasts, and our hearts. It will also deal with diet and exercise, accidents in the home, hysterectomies, and whether or not we can trust the health studies. Some of the other essays include discussions on longevity, medical directives, the body/mind connection, physical disabilities, hearing loss, vision, and those all-powerful hormones.

Consider the Source

"I am being hit from all sides with things I must do, foods I must eat, ways I must think to stay forever young. I get exhausted just thinking about it."

—Hila Colman, "Just Desserts," *New York Times Magazine* (May 3, 1998)

Susan Calvert Finn, Ph.D., author of *Women's Nutrition for Healthy Living*, says that when we evaluate health information, we should consider the source. She suggests we "check who funded the research if results benefit a particular food or drug. Also consider the study subjects. Animal research may not apply to people, and research on men or women may not apply to the other sex. Always look for multiple studies on the same topic."

Consider the source. Look for multiple studies on the same topic. Many of us in midlife and beyond don't have the time to fool around with research at the library or on the Internet (and whom do you believe there?) to access multiple studies on the use of yogurt spread versus the spread made with soy milk. I'm busy playing with my grandchildren. Is jelly made from organically grown red currants better for me than Smuckers? I just want to eat my toast in peace. Whom do we believe? What about my cholesterol? What about my colon? Fiber, fat, sugar, phytoestrogens, nutritional supplements, herbs, high blood pressure. Whom do we trust? One day I'm supposed to be eating one thing, drinking another. Next day the news report says I have it backwards—or do they? Consider the source.

I'll pay attention to the studies, but I'm also going to start listening to *me*. From this day forward I am going to pay attention to the body and the intuition I've been given. I reside in a wise, finely tuned instrument that knows (if I listen) when I'm abusing it, and it lets me know.

How do you feel about this?

_____

_____

_____

_____

The Next Fifty Years

What can you do to listen more carefully to your body?

_____

_____

_____

_____

Yoga and Yogurt

"I tried doing just yoga and eating yogurt to lose weight and I felt like a starving pretzel."

—Mary Alice, 67

Unfortunately, society makes it a lot easier to go wild with a credit card or to throw down a few glasses of fine wine than to start a painting, meditating, or doing yoga. Acquisition and speed are highly valued in our culture, and we expect our activities to have a clear purpose.

I've been very attracted to yoga in the past few years, mainly because the only gear you need is a towel, loose-fitting clothing, and clean socks without holes. And I had read that the Delany sisters, who lived to be well over 100, did some yoga stretches every day.

So one day I found myself sitting cross-legged on the orange-carpeted floor of a yoga center in my town. I was feeling optimistic and nervous. Although this was a beginning yoga class, the students around me, all older women, exuded a confidence in their bodies I knew I wanted to have. I started out feeling meditative as a Buddha, and when I glanced in the mirror, I saw I actually looked like one! Belly protruding, look of serenity on my face. I watched as one of the younger women in her forties lay down on the floor and brought her legs over her head. Buddha or not, I was not attempting that one.

What is yoga? The word itself is derived from the word "yoke" in Sanskrit. Does that tell you something? It's a mind/body discipline that was developed in India some 5,000 years ago. Hatha yoga is a series of slow, deliberate poses that enhance flexibility, improve circulation, and increase concentration.

Pleasure is the real reason I practice yoga. The need for exercise and flexibility got me to sign up for the class. But I returned again and again for something else. During the class, the ego disappears—the me who measures her body against all the other women, and the me who worries about her $3,000 credit card debt. The ego evaporates and the biography society writes about us disappears. What is left? It's hard to explain, but it feels like my truest self.

How do you feel about this?

_____

_____

_____

_____

What are you willing to do to help your body feel peaceful and flexible?

_____

_____

_____

_____

Food Is My Friend

"I've never had any problem with cholesterol. As we say at the American Institute of Wine and Food, 'Small helpings, no seconds, a little bit of everything, no snacking and have a good time.'"

—Julia Child

At this point in your life you don't need me to tell you that regardless of how much you weigh, your metabolism has likely slowed down. Simply put, if you don't modify your eating habits to accommodate this change in metabolism, you'll gain weight.

Grandma always said, "You are what you eat." She lived to be 101. Funny, she didn't look like a steak cooked in butter, a baked potato with sour cream, and pudding with fresh whipped cream. I read somewhere that "inside some of us is a thin person struggling to get out, but she can usually be sedated with a few pieces of chocolate cake." Should we eat cake? When I was traveling through Massachusetts some years ago, I read in the *Worcester Telegram and Gazette* that Mary Marques, 104, of Palmer, Massachusetts, was honored in Boston, along with seven other centenarians. She attributed her longevity to eating lots of vegetables and drinking a glass of red wine every day. No mention of cake!

I used to eat apple pie for breakfast, fettuccini alfredo for lunch, mashed potatoes and gravy for dinner, tiramisu for dessert—who would want to change that menu?! Yet I turned 50 and the pounds were packing on faster than I could count them.

I've become agitated in my quest to decipher which advice I should follow. Yesterday I tripped and nearly fell trying to find my glasses so I could read the nutritional information on the cereal box. And if I become agitated, that gets in the way of my feeling peaceful, and constant agitation is bad for your health (so is falling down). Help! I'm caught in a sticky web of multiple nutritional studies and funded research. I'm getting a migraine from surfing the National Institute for Health web site. Maybe the radiation from the computer screen is a health hazard. Maybe looking up web sites on what's healthy is unhealthy for me.

One study says apple juice is a cholesterol fighter. Apple juice contains one of the best sources of cholesterol-fighting phenols. Phenols are plant compounds that protect the arteries from the adverse effects of "bad" LDL cholesterol. And guess what? Some other good phenol sources are cranberry juice, apples, red grapes or red grape juice, and red wine.

Consider rejecting processed fare that is high in fat or sweeteners in favor of unprocessed, fiber-rich whole grains and produce; these foods, besides meeting our nutritional needs, may send a stronger signal to the brain that we've eaten enough.

And ladies, dining out shouldn't mean deprivation if you're trying to eat healthfully. What you eat is not as important as *how much* you eat. To control portion size, just request a half portion or one to share, and ask for a doggy bag. Leftovers are great for lunch the next day.

Women can reduce their risk of heart disease by almost 30 percent by eating two to three servings of whole grains a day, and it's easy to get those servings into your diet. Try a cup of oatmeal for breakfast and a sandwich on whole wheat bread for lunch. Or have brown rice instead of white with dinner and a cup of popcorn at snack time.

We now have supermarkets full of low-fat yogurt, whole-grain bagels, and precut vegetables, so following a healthy diet can be as simple as steering your grocery cart down one or two aisles and skipping the rest.

Your body is trying to tell you something important every day. Listen. Trust that your body knows how much fuel it needs for the day—you don't have to eat every meal! As we age, our sense of taste diminishes, so make everything you eat look beautiful.

What's a woman to do? As author Barbara Holland said in *Wasn't the Grass Greener?*, "Day before yesterday alcohol was poison, yesterday a couple of drinks improved the heart, today they'll be the death of us. Tuesday eggs were the staff of life; Wednesday they were lethal."

Okay, let's be rational. Today I will only worry about today. I will eat foods that are healthy for me—the ones I learned about in home economics 48 years ago. You know, the pyramid diagram with the fish and eggs, the dairy products, grains, etc. That's what I'll do today. And if I eat something that doesn't feel good in my body, I'll put that on the list of items I won't be eating again soon.

How do you feel about this?

_____

_____

_____

_____

What changes can you make in your diet that will help you feel healthy and maintain a healthy weight?

_____

_____

_____

_____

The Longevity Test

"Life is like a great jazz riff. You sense the end the very moment you were wanting it to go on forever."

—Sheila Ballantyne, writer

Today I took the longevity test in *Living to 100: Lessons in Living to Your Maximum Potential at Any Age* by Thomas T. Perls et al.

My calculations tell me I could live to be 95 in fairly good health. Some of the factors that will help me do this are "yes" answers to: Do you drink a glass of red wine daily (+2)? Do you avoid the sun and use sunblock (+3)? Can you shed stress (+7)? Yes, it sounds like sitting peacefully in the shade with a glass of red wine is the way to go (or the way to live—I don't mean "go" in the dead sense).

Now I'm thinking about what it means to live until I'm 95. At this writing I'm 56, and according to the test I've got approximately 40 more years as a resident of this planet. Decisions must be made and I'm full of disturbing questions.

Do I get the chance to retire with my husband? Will we instead suffer the loss or illness of one of us, which would change the entire picture? Is it safe to make a plan knowing that going it alone is a possibility? Am I doing all I can do to stay healthy? Am I making the right decisions about healthcare? I say, make a plan and if you need to change it you will. If you are meant to face life on your own, then you will make some hard decisions and go on living your remaining years. I say, guarantees are not what life is about and it's still worth living.

Today I took the longevity test and I wasn't given a guarantee of living all the way to 95. In spite of that, I plan to do some amazing things no matter how much time and how challenging the circumstances I'll have to face in the years ahead.

How do you feel about this?

_____

_____

_____

_____

What challenges do you see yourself overcoming in the years ahead?

_____

_____

_____

_____

_____

_____

_____

Why Should I Exercise!?

"I exercise with a stationary bike and a thing called a rickshaw. And every day, I walk about one-half mile to and from the restaurant at the retirement community for breakfast."

—Julia Child, at age 90, in *Bottom Line Personal* (September 2002)

Let me assure you, I'm not an exercise guru or gym queen. I eat well and take daily vitamin supplements. I drag myself to the gym or up onto my treadmill in front of the TV with consistent irregularity. I'm not trying to measure up to the media standards of the sleek, sweaty, rippling woman pumping away on the step machine. After three children (one a Caesarian) I don't have any fantasies of having a washboard stomach. Basic maintenance and slowing the inevitable decline are my goals.

A well-developed exercise program not only reshapes and trims your body, it decreases your chances of heart attacks, osteoporosis, certain types of arthritis, and other conditions that creep up on us in our middle and later years. For me, one of exercise's most valuable outcomes is the increase in my body's level of endorphins—those valuable chemicals that produce an emotional high. Creating a steady supply of endorphins through regular exercise can do more for our bodies and our mental health during menopause and beyond than all the cosmetics and plastic surgery in the world.

Exercise can prolong your life regardless of heredity. A Finnish study tracked 16,000 adult twins for 19 years, and the active twin had a much lower chance of dying prematurely. According to the study, people who walked briskly, jogged, or did an equivalent exercise for 30 minutes at least six times a month had more than a 40 percent lower death rate than those who were sedentary.

It is almost never too late to improve your physical condition and performance. Every year, more and more women ages 50 to 90-plus compete in sports such as track and field, swimming, volleyball, and archery. These athletes are exceeding expectations of what was previously considered possible. Fan Benno-Caris, 82-year-old award-winning racewalker and international intuitive counselor who was interviewed for Cynthia Black's book *Our Turn, Our Time: Women Truly Coming of Age*, said, "I plan to win the World Games eighteen years from now. I'll be one hundred years young, and I invite you all to be there."

Walking makes us smarter. A study of sedentary seniors aged 60 to 65 found that those who walked briskly for 15 to 45 minutes three times a week improved their performance on computer-related tasks, compared with those who did one hour of stretching and toning three times weekly. It is thought that the extra flow of oxygen to the brain promoted by walking slows age-related decline in mental functioning. Women over 50 who stay active in activities such as sports, board games, painting, and gardening are much less likely to contract Alzheimer's later in life.

Women today have so many exercise machines and classes to choose from. After checking with your doctor, pick one or two exercises that you like. The best exercise is the one you will continue to do regularly because it feels good. To stay motivated, we must each ask ourselves why we want to be fit. My response is that I want to maintain my muscular strength and balance so I won't become too dependent in my later years. I also want to have the physical and mental energy to travel and to do things with my grandchildren.

How do you feel about this?

_____

_____

_____

_____

What do you want from life that would motivate you to start an exercise program or to stay with the one you already have in place?

_____

_____

_____

_____

Where Are My Glasses!?

"I am still surprised when I need my spectacles to read a menu or scan the telephone directory."

—Melody Beattie, *Journey to the Heart*

It used to be that my glasses were never where I was when I needed them. Now, I have ten-dollar drugstore half-frame magnifying glasses (150+ diopter) placed all over my house. I love them so much that when one of the "arms" breaks off, I don't throw them out. One pair with a broken arm hangs over the edge of the reading materials bin in the master bath. Another stands in the pencil cup in the kitchen for reading recipes, the ingredients list on the back of packaged foods, and the label on my vitamins. Question: How come the "take as directed" information on the back of my 50-plus nutritional supplements is written in a typeface that only someone under 30 could read?

I'll never forget the time I was sitting across from one of my clients, who gave me something to read. When I couldn't find my glasses I got up and excused myself, saying I needed to go hunt down my glasses. Before I could get out of my office my client rather shyly said, "Dr. Blair, you've got several pairs on you already." When I looked I had one pair tucked in the V neck of my sweater, and two pairs, one behind the other, perched on my head.

If you keep losing your glasses like I do, try attaching a strip of Velcro to your glasses case and the corresponding strip to your reading chair or nightstand and stick them on. Wear your glasses attached to a chain or cord hung around your neck. When you take them off, hang them on a hook you've installed near your desk or reading chair.

There are four common age-related vision problems. Fortunately, they can be helped. That's why it's important to get your eyes checked regularly even if you don't notice any problems.

- presbyopia—reading-distance vision changes by about age 40
- macular degeneration—central vision deteriorates
- glaucoma—peripheral vision blurs
- cataract—eye lens grows cloudy and vision blurs or dims

One doctor advises that starting as early as 30, you should begin vision screening for cataracts and retinal vascular degeneration. Another says eat four servings per week of dark green leafy vegetables, such as spinach, kale, and collard greens, which have been shown to protect against such degeneration.

There are benefits to not seeing as well as I did in my younger years. My house always looks dust free and my wrinkles are harder to see. Someone once said, "If you really don't want to worry about aging, just don't put your glasses on when you look in the mirror."

How do you feel about this?

_____

_____

_____

_____

When was the last time you had your eyes checked? Do you need a new pair of glasses? A new prescription?

_____

_____

_____

_____

What You Don't "No" Can Hurt You

"You just realize that you are a very finite creature and that you must do what you want and finish out your appointed tasks—and learn to say 'no' more."

—Gail Goodwin, *Fabulous Friends*

The exciting thing about being in midlife and older is that nature gives you another chance to live life on your terms. Saying no to the things that zap your energy will leave you time for the things that bring you fulfillment and happiness. Learn to say no without guilt. If you don't, you end up doing things you don't want to or shouldn't be doing—all the while acting, on the surface, as if everything is just fine. In *I am a Woman Finding My Voice*, Janet Quinn says, "More and more, I am claiming the fullness of my right to choose; I am celebrating my freedom to be a woman saying NO!"

Is someone in your life asking you to do something that compromises your self-respect or integrity or just doesn't feel right? Would fulfilling the other person's need take away from your sense of well-being? Does that person's request come at a bad time so that it detracts from your health and happiness? Are you in a pattern in which you are doing for, or giving to others but getting very little in return?

I suggest you develop a habit of saying, "Let me think about it and I'll get back to you." Ask yourself, "All things considered, is it in my best interest to says yes, or is it okay to refuse?" Don't say yes right away to every request. It's okay to say I need a few minutes, hours, or days to think about this. But remember that you are not making the other person wrong for asking you something. You are simply standing up for your own needs.

When you start learning to say no, you'll have to deal with the other person's reaction, which could range from anger to downright lack of acceptance of your position. Stick to your guns. If you don't, you will ultimately lose respect for yourself or build up huge resentments.

As older, wiser women we need to say a clear and definite *yes* to some uses of our time and a resounding *no* to others. You need time that you regularly set aside without apology or explanation; time not easily given over to compromise. It's all right to putter, to spend time without any need to achieve.

Our culture conditions us as young girls to please others, and it doesn't take a little girl very long to realize that people-pleasing and self-sacrifice are a way to gain self-worth. As a result, you may often feel guilty when you get up the courage to say no to others who request your time and attention.

How do you feel about this?

_____

_____

_____

_____

Can you think of someone or something you need to start saying "no" to?

_____

_____

_____

_____

What Did You Say?

"Maybe the reason our hearing diminishes after age 50 is because there are just some things we don't want to hear anymore. Like you're too old to roller skate!"

—Alison, 59

In talking about her loss of hearing in old age, Helen Hayes said in her autobiography, "Fighting as hard as we can against a disability is essential; we don't want to give in and give up. But denying it, for reasons of pride or prejudice, is a whole other matter."

It's a fact of life that as you mature, some of your sensory abilities will weaken, and hearing loss is accepted by many as a normal part of aging. About half of women over 65 have some degree of hearing loss but most don't know it. In fact, hearing loss ranks with heart disease as one of the most common physical problems. The most common type of hearing loss is associated with aging, but because it occurs gradually, in many cases it goes unnoticed for years. Early detection is important for effective treatment.

Warning signs include: voices get lost in background noise, you favor one ear, you get ringing or buzzing in the ears, you wonder why everyone is mumbling, you turn up the TV or radio volume until others complain, you need to look at people to understand what they're saying, and you may become socially withdrawn and avoid initiating conversations.

Can't hear but don't want a clunky hearing aid? Get over it! Options now include in-the-ear, in-the-canal (less conspicuous), and completely-in-the-canal (unnoticeable) models, in addition to behind-the-ear devices. An audiologist can help you find the right fit for your ear, your particular kind of hearing loss, and your budget. Many new hearing aids are now digital instead of analog; the result is better reproduction of incoming sounds and an improved ability to handle background noise. Some even use an artificial intelligence system to distinguish speech from noise, and microchips so small they fit in the eye of a needle. There is something new under the sun every day, it seems.

Ask for a simple hearing test from your physician or a certified audiologist before symptoms arise. And remember, a hearing aid can greatly improve even a minor hearing loss.

How do you feel about this?

_____

_____

_____

_____

_____

Describe your particular hearing loss (if any) and take this info your doctor:

_____

_____

_____

_____

Uteruses and Vaginas

"I can't stand how grim everyone is about aging—
osteoporosis, liver spots, vaginal dryness—oh, please!"

—Valerie Harper, *Today I Am a Ma'am*

Let's face it. If you're an older women, you have at least a vagina and maybe a uterus. These precious body parts deserve our attention just like any other body part. I'll start this discussion with our friend the vagina (Mom used to refer to it as "down there").

When women enter menopause, one of the most common complaints is vaginal dryness during sex, which can make intercourse feel scratchy or painful. Fortunately, medical science has come to the rescue. Talk to your gynecologist regarding prescriptions, lubricants, hormone creams that can thicken and nourish the vaginal tissues. You may also want to try a nonhormonal lubricant.

Here's another place where exercise can help. Regular toning of your vaginal muscles increases circulation to this area of your body and helps keep vaginal tissues moist and healthy. Exercise your vaginal muscles by doing Kegel exercises. Squeeze your vaginal muscles (these are the same ones you use to stop the flow of urine) and hold them for ten seconds and relax. Repeat several times per day. I do them whenever I'm stopped at a traffic light or in line at the supermarket. As you're doing these discreet exercises, try not to contract your thighs, buttocks, or abdominals at the same time, and visualize "down there" as healthy, pink, moist, and resilient.

Now for your uterus. If you still have a uterus, you may be one of the 40 percent of U.S. women who have uterine fibroids. Some fibroids go away of their own accord, while others stay and cause problems. Although there are dietary and hormonal reasons that so many women have these growths, the baseline energetic causes of fibroids may have to do with blockage and stagnation of the energy of the pelvis. In her widely acclaimed newsletter called *Health Wisdom for Women*, Dr. Christiane Northrup suggests that "the illnesses that originate in this area of the body are activated by prolonged stress from fear of losing control over our physical environments. . . . Fibroids represent creative energy that hasn't been birthed. We are at risk for fibroids when we direct our energy into any dead-end relationship . . . a job, a marriage, a family or virtually any situation that is less than fulfilling."

If you've had a hysterectomy or are anticipating one, remember that a hysterectomy doesn't necessarily diminish your sexuality. Most women who have hysterectomies report more sexual activity and greater pleasure after the operation than before it. The probable reason—the symptoms that usually lead to hysterectomy, including pain and heavy bleeding, keep women from enjoying sex fully before the operation.

So, pay attention to those parts "down there" so you can get on with living. How do you feel about this?

_____

_____

_____

_____

Is there anything you need to discuss with your gynecologist?

_____

_____

_____

_____

Sleeping

"In an ordinary year . . . one out of four hundred Americans will be injured just lying in bed, generally because of the headboard collapsing, the frame giving way, or some other mechanical failure."

—Barbara Johnson, *Living Somewhere between Estrogen and Death*

Just like air, food, and water, sleep is a basic necessity. Some researchers say that lack of sleep may make you age faster. The lack seems to affect carbohydrate metabolism and endocrine function, which are effects that normally occur with aging. The research suggests that sleep deprivation may increase the severity of disorders related to age.

On the other hand, don't worry if you don't get eight hours sleep a night. Sleep habits are almost as individual as handwriting. There's no medical necessity that everyone get eight hours sleep. The unbroken, sound sleep of youth is a thing of the past for most older women. Doctors say this is a normal change with age. It's neither good nor bad, but this change worries many women when it shouldn't.

As for snoring, nothing seems to affect an otherwise happy relationship like the rumble of a freight train coming from the pillow next to you. I think sleeping in separate beds can help a relationship, especially if your partner is snoring. The objective is to have as healthy a relationship as possible when awake. If sleeping separately improves the daytime relationship, then do it.

Chronic lack of sleep can make nonsnoring partners irritable, affect concentration and judgment, and even harm a marriage. We may become angry at them, but snorers have no control over their noisemaking, and it may be a sign of obstructive sleep apnea, a serious threat to health. Instead of getting angry, encourage them to seek medical help.

If you or your mate is snoring, here are some things you can do:

- Lose weight to get rid of excess, flabby tissue in the throat.
- Don't drink anything containing alcohol for three to four hours before sleep.
- If you have nasal congestion ask your doctor about using a decongestant/antihistamine.
- Use adhesive nasal strips to hold your nostrils open.
- Raise up the head of your bed about four inches, or get an orthopedic pillow with rolls that will support your neck and pull your chin up.
- Stop smoking—it can irritate the airways, worsening snoring.
- Avoid sedative-type medications, such as sleeping pills and tranquilizers.
- Humidify the bedroom.
- Learn to sleep on your side; sleeping on your back increases snoring.
- Avoid heavy snacks before bed.

Snoring aside, here are some helpful tips for getting a good night's sleep:

- Establish a regular bedtime schedule.
- Create a comfortable bed. Buy a good mattress and comfy sheets.
- Exercise regularly, but not for two or three hours before bedtime.
- Make your bedroom conducive to sleep.

- Keep your bedroom at an optimal temperature and noise level.
- Relax and take a bubble bath.
- Do yoga, listen to peaceful music, or meditate.
- Do some light reading.
- Leave your worries behind. Write them down in a journal and close it.
- Set regular times for sleeping and waking, and try not to vary from the schedule.
- Avoid caffeine, alcohol, and tobacco products before bedtime.
- Don't eat a lot, but have a light snack so hunger doesn't keep you up.

How are you sleeping these days?

_____

_____

_____

_____

What things can you do to create a better night's sleep?

_____

_____

_____

_____

Physical Disability

"When I can see my brokenness with the eyes of compassion instead of judgment, I heal and become more compassionate with the brokenness of others. Healing always happens when I choose to remember to be a woman being gentle with myself."

—Janet F. Quinn, *I Am a Woman Finding My Voice*

I intend to work on this book today, so I "run" around the house collecting pen, paper, and more coffee to take out to the backyard. Of course, I make the mistake of listening to the answering machine, which distracts me for a while. I will set up on the back patio and write. I will light a fire in my outdoor fireplace and elevate my feet by placing them on a small plastic coffee table. Write and drink coffee.

I'm not exactly "running" these days. I've opted to have my painful bunions corrected. Bunion—sounds like a funny vegetable. A cross between an onion and bump, but it's actually a serious foot deformity, a misalignment of bones. The surgery, called a bunionectomy, was for me an agonizing, fear-inducing adventure. On the operating table the surgeon makes a seven-inch incision, slices open the "bumpy onion," takes out a couple of hunks of bone, inserts a screw and two wires to keep the newly formed foot in place, sews you up, sends you off in a clunky, splinted boot cast with Velcro closings, and tells you not to put any weight on your toes: "Walk on your heel, keep the foot elevated, take these painkillers when you need them, see you in a week, the cast stays on for a month."

Tomorrow I will have my first shower in days. I imagine it will be a humbling experience. My husband will assist me: he'll wrap the cast in garbage bags and get a good look at my cellulite legs and blubbery bottom as he positions me in the shower, standing by in case I slip and fall. I imagine I'll feel like a child again—or an old, old lady dependent on a home healthcare aide for all necessary body care and maintenance.

I imagine I will be grateful that I have a husband to help care for me. I imagine what it would be like without one—alone and needing paid strangers to come into my home, viewing my cellulite. I imagine what it would be like to live in a country without doctors who do this kind of surgery. I imagine what it would be like not to have the option to correct my foot because I lacked insurance or resources.

So, I'm trying not to be distracted by the throbbing pain, stinging incision, and swelling going on underneath the bandages. I'm trying not to be a whiny baby, a spoiled brat. I'm trying to count my blessings. As I fantasize throwing my cast into the fire, I lower a too large log into the backyard fireplace to warm up the cool morning, then with flames leaping and wood sputtering, I hobble back to my comfy outdoor sofa, put my foot up, stare up at the gentle swaying red maple bowing over me, birds singing in the branches, and realize how lucky I am today to be alive and on the mend.

How do you feel about this?

Heart Health

"You have double the risk of having a heart attack for two hours after getting angry!"

—Mary Ann Mayo

Bet you didn't know that marital difficulties can increase a woman's risk of heart attack. A woman who has had a heart attack or other acute cardiac episode, and whose marital difficulties include substance abuse, infidelity, economic difficulties, or partner's illness, is more likely to suffer another episode. Women are twice as likely as men to die after one heart attack and are more likely to have a second heart attack within four years. Have I scared you enough?

Here are some interesting heart facts that I've collected from a wide variety of reliable sources:

1. According to nutritionists, chocolate is good for your heart. Studies show that one ounce of dark chocolate contains ten times more antioxidants than one ounce of strawberries. Even better, a diet that includes one ounce of chocolate per day seems to increase HDL (that's the "good" cholesterol) and to prevent LDL ("bad" cholesterol) from oxidizing—one of the possible contributing factors for heart disease. If the extra calories and sugar aren't a problem, chocolate can be part of a healthy diet! Isn't that amazing?

2. One study showed that one cup of black tea a day was enough to lower heart attack risk by 44 percent.

3. Heart attacks are seasonal. They peak during December and January, when there are 33 percent more deaths from heart attacks than in summer and early fall. The reasons could be increased food, alcohol, and salt consumption; additional stress; respiratory infections; and reduced hours of daylight.

4. Women who heed the exhortations to eat nutritious meals, exercise daily, and not smoke could reduce their risk of heart disease by 82 percent.

The *Journal of the American Heart Association* says *always* call 911 if you feel you are having a heart attack. The average heart attack sufferer usually waits about two hours before seeking medical attention. The faster you get to the hospital, the better your chances are for successful treatment. They have found that delays are significantly longer among homemakers, non-Hispanic blacks, elderly people, disabled people, and Medicaid recipients. So have your doctor explain the symptoms of cardiac trouble, so you can recognize a potential heart attack quickly. And by all means, check with your doctor about taking an aspirin upon the onset of any troubling symptoms.

The American Heart Association tells us that women's symptoms of heart attack are not the same as those for men. Women may experience chest, stomach, or abdominal pain that does not necessarily feel acute or crushing, nausea or dizziness, shortness of breath, heart palpitations, fatigue, or a general feeling of weakness. Doctors recommend that if you are having symptoms of heart attack, you should chew a full-strength aspirin and get to the hospital ASAP.

These days, having heart disease is not an automatic death sentence, it's a call to action. A time to make changes for a long and vigorous life. A time to get off the couch and discover the joy of living. Furthermore, optimistic people who have had heart attacks are less likely to suffer subsequent heart problems, and their recovery is almost three times faster.

How do you feel about this?

_____

_____

_____

_____

What steps can you take starting today to protect your heart?

_____

_____

_____

_____

Healing Pets

*"Animals are our spiritual companions, living proof
of a simply abundant source of love."*

—Sarah Ban Breathnach, *Simple Abundance*

In *It's Better to Be over the Hill Than Under It*, Eda LeShan writes that "holding the warm body of a cat that is purring is a kind of special contact that begins to evaporate from our lives as we become widowed and children and grandchildren move far away and nobody has time for hugs." This "special contact" has clearly established medical and emotional benefits.

In the last two decades, scientists have discovered that the bond we form with pets can make an enormous difference to our health—sometimes the difference between life and death. Research reveals that pet owners are less likely than people without pets to develop heart disease and that pet owners who have heart attacks live longer than coronary attack victims without pets. Studies show that pet owners of all ages go to their doctors less often, have more fun, and feel more secure than those who have no pets. Experts tell us that pets like dogs and cats can help control blood pressure, and some studies show that a pet's calming influence is better at controlling high blood pressure than antihypertension drugs.

Nursing homes report that when they bring animals into their environments, patient death rates drop by an amazing 40 percent and the need for medication decreases. Research has shown that the presence of pet birds reduced the depression and loneliness in elderly people hospitalized or in old-age homes.

If you don't want the long-term commitment of a pet or can't afford to own one, you can take advantage of a wonderful volunteer opportunity through your local animal shelter or humane society. If you are willing to commit to a two- to six-week situation, you can be a foster parent for a lost or rescued pet needing a place to stay while they recover from a minor illness or because they are too young yet for adoption.

One 64-year-old woman I spoke with said, "On days when my arthritis is acting up, my little dog gives me a reason to cope. I have to take care of him so I get up and do things for him and he loves me back." In *The Last Gift of Time: Life beyond Sixty*, Carolyn G. Heilbrun writes, "No one who has not, upon returning from any absence, long or short, been greeted by a loving dog

The Next Fifty Years

can understand what devotion is." Whether it's the need for affection, company, or health, consider bringing a pet into your life.

How do you feel about this topic?

_____

_____

_____

_____

If you don't already have a pet, what kind of pet do you see yourself with in the future (if any)?

_____

Don't Fall Down!

"Each year, one-third of people over age 65 take a tumble. . . . Most falls are not random or an inevitable part of aging."

—Margaret Gottschalk, Yale-New Haven Hospital

I live in a house that was built in 1928. As opposed to modern houses where the washer and dryer are more conveniently located, my machines are down a flight of wooden stairs ending in a poured concrete basement floor. I've been thinking more and more about how it would feel to fall down those stairs (or up them) with no one around to see or hear me tumble. With this in mind, I have vowed to keep up my strength and balance exercises and I try to remember to clip my cell phone to my belt whenever I go down the basement stairs just in case.

Balance problems may strike more frequently after age 50, but you can counteract the problems associated with balance by doing some simple exercises. Ask a personal trainer. Most falls by seniors at home are not caused by household hazards but by weak muscles, in addition to bad eyesight (I avoid walking in my bifocals) and poorly constructed shoes. Very few falls are associated with common potential hazards, such as loose rugs and slippery bathtubs.

The best way for us to avoid falls is to strengthen muscles, improve balance, preserve vision, wear appropriate footwear, monitor the effects of medication, and remove potential hazards.

Also, many medications can cause drowsiness or affect blood pressure causing dizziness. When getting out of bed or rising from a chair, do so slowly. If you're prone to dizziness, ask the doctor to check for something called "postural hypotension."

Health and age-related changes that contribute to falls include arthritis and decreased sensation in the feet, known as peripheral neuropathy. The other major cause of falls is hazardous conditions in the home environment. Fortunately, there are numerous ways to reduce these hazards for yourself or a loved one. Many of them involve little or no cost.

Keep floors clear of small objects, avoid waxing floors, and remove loose wires; scatter rugs are dangerous, stairways should be well lit, night lights are a must in the bathroom. Wear shoes that provide solid support. As you walk down stairs, go slowly and keep at least one hand free to hold the railing. Take off your reading glasses when walking around, and always keep your regular glasses clean. Eliminate throw rugs. Don't highly polish your floors. Put secure bars in the bathroom along with a bright night light. If you fall repeatedly, you might look into something they sell called "hip protectors" to decrease the impact of a fall on the hip and reduce the risk of fracture.

In the kitchen keep the pots, dishes, and staple foods you use regularly within easy reach. Store the heaviest items in the lower cupboards. If you must reach high places, get a step stool that has a high handrail and rubber tips. Never use a chair.

In the bedroom keep a lamp within easy reach of your bed and a flashlight on hand in case there's a power failure. Keep a phone at your bedside. If your bedroom doesn't have a phone jack, get a cordless phone and keep the receiver with you at night.

Keep the path clear from your bed to the bathroom.

Have someone install grab bars by the toilet and in the bathtub or shower area if you need them. Use a rubber mat with suction cups in the tub or shower, and a nonskid bath mat on the floor. Consider a bathtub seat or shower chair and a handheld shower head so you can shower sitting down. Buy a raised toilet seat if you have trouble getting on and off the toilet.

On your stairwells make sure the steps are in good repair and have a nonskid surface with solid handrails on both sides of stairways. Keep steps free of clutter. Make sure the stairwells are well lit.

The Next Fifty Years

As time goes on, you may want to sign on with a personal emergency response service, whereby you wear a small, lightweight, waterproof pendant or bracelet that has a button to press if you run into trouble or fall. If balance becomes an ongoing problem, consider a cane or walker.

Above all, the most important action to take to prevent falling is some regular exercise. Older women participating in regular exercise may suffer fewer injuries from falls, as weight training increases bone density and reaction time.

How do you feel about this?

_____

_____

_____

_____

What steps are you willing to take to help prevent falls in your home and when you're out in public?

_____

_____

_____

_____

Coffee and the Pee-Pee Dance

"Bladder control problems should not be looked upon either as an inevitable part of aging or as a disease, but rather as a problem that can be managed and possibly corrected if you are determined to do so."

—Paula B. Doress-Worters and Diana L. Siegal, *The New Ourselves, Growing Older*

An AARP magazine article said that coffee lovers should rejoice. They've discovered that older women who were lifetime java drinkers beat their peers in 11 out of 12 tests of mental abilities in a recent study. It turns out that the caffeine may offset some types of age-related mental decline.

Well, it's nice that someone discovered we can increase our mental abilities by drinking coffee. But, I ask you, does that increased mental ability assist you in making all those trips to the bathroom? And what about the trips to the bathroom that you don't quite make? Have you ever done the pee-pee dance or the cross-legged bunny hop on your way to relieve yourself?

If you're a coffee lover, you probably enjoy stopping for a nice hot cup at a diner while you're on an extended car trip, only to regret it 30 minutes later. Have you ever sped into a gas station, left the car running, jumped out, and dashed to the ladies' room only to find the door locked? One time I nearly knocked someone over in the station's food mart while grabbing for the key suspended by a wood block beside the cash register.

You can ask your doctor or gynecologist about medication to help you with this issue. Or you can cut down on your coffee consumption. I'm drinking green tea these days. They say green tea helps with many aging and health issues. My morning coffee is now a half and half mix of caffeinated and decaffeinated coffees. And when I'm on the road, I avoid coffee and sodas with caffeine altogether.

Now you'll need to decide. Mental ability or wet pants? Maybe you don't have to choose. Make some small changes and you can still enjoy your occasional cup of coffee without having to do the pee-pee dance or mop the floor on the way to the bathroom.

How do you feel about this?

_____

_____

_____

_____

When considering this issue, what small changes can you make?

_____

_____

_____

_____

Chew on This

"One charming grande dame . . . claims she copes with her failing memory by feeling her toothbrush before she brushes her teeth. If it's wet . . . she knows she's already done that."

—Frances Weaver, *The Girls with the Grandmother Faces*

Boy, was I surprised to find out that I needed periodontal work done. Gum disease. Furthermore, I needed to have surgery—cut and sew my gums. Yikes! Thank God for nitrous oxide (laughing gas). Have I scared you enough? Sorry. But this is important, and I have to get your attention. The good news is, flossing helps and regular deep-cleaning in the dentist's chair can take care of it. However, some of us (like me) have simply inherited weak gums.

One positive trend among the aging population is the increasing attention to dental and oral health. Surveys, like one done for the federal government and the American Dental Association, indicate that a greater percentage of seniors are making regular visits to the dentist. However, despite the improvements, problems remain. A report from the Department of Health and Human Services found that one-third of seniors with natural teeth have untreated dental cavities in their crowns or roots. Bummer!

So, let me say it again—floss. See your dentist regularly. Have your teeth deep-cleaned at least once a year. You'll improve the odds of keeping your own teeth into very old age, and wouldn't that be nice? I've read that keeping your gums healthy could even prevent a heart attack. Evidently, periodontal disease is a risk factor for cardiovascular problems.

I'm sorry I scared you a bit, but if you want to eat more than applesauce and oatmeal in your later years, take good care of your teeth and gums.

How do you feel about this?

_____

_____

_____

_____

What steps can you take to improve your oral health?

_____

_____

_____

_____

Breasts

"This last and significant passage of my life, my aging, deserves my full attention and devotion."

—Ruth Raymond Thone, *Women and Aging: Celebrating Ourselves*

Breast cancer is a big fear in older women and although 90 percent of us will never develop it, there is still every reason in the world to protect yourself as best you can. Okay, maybe you go for your mammogram according to the recommended schedule. But maybe you don't. Or if you do, you dread it. Maybe you resist going because it's so uncomfortable, like having your breasts slammed between two large encyclopedias in a machine invented by men.

Here's some information that may ease your anxiety. I recently found out about something called a "comfort pad." This thin foam rubber pad attaches to the metal squeeze plates and comes in various sizes to accommodate most women. The result is a much more tolerable exam. Not every mammogram facility offers these wonderful pads, but do take the time to ask if they have them available. When I asked the technician about them, she had to dig a box of pads out from somewhere in the back of a storage closet. She said most people don't know about them. When the pressure of those steel plates was applied—ahhh, what a relief. Still some discomfort, but much less.

Some of you have probably experienced a lump or have been treated for breast cancer. Please nag the rest of us to take our breast health seriously. You've been there. We'll listen to you. Tell your story to every woman who will listen. Offer to go with someone who is fearful. You may just help save a life.

How do you feel about this?

_____

_____

_____

_____

What are you willing to do to promote your breast health or that of someone else?

_____

_____

_____

_____

Medical Directives

*"It bothers me that someone else might have
to make decisions for me . . . but, it's also a
comfort knowing someone I've chosen would
speak for me when I can't speak for myself."*

—Joan, 71

The AARP suggests we have a plan in place, just in case "stuff happens."
Considering and implementing what they suggest may bring up denial and
avoidance. It did for me. Who wants to think and plan ahead for the worst?
Then again, I imagine myself in a coma trying to kick myself because I hadn't
done anything to put some important medical directives down on paper.

So here's what I did. I did one of the things on the list of suggestions below
every month or so. It took me about a year to put it all in place because it emotionally overloaded me. Denial and avoidance. Now I'm glad I got it done.

• Discuss your wishes with family members, doctors, and caregivers.
• Consult an attorney about a living will.
• Avoid generic advance directive forms; compile and update documents
  with your doctor's input.

- Pick a healthcare agent or proxy who will act aggressively on your behalf; the person closest to you may not always be the best.
- Sign each directive, date it, and have it witnessed according to the laws in your state.
- Put copies of your advance directives in your medical records and make them widely available to family and care providers.

My advice to you, put a plan in place and get on with living.

How do you feel about this?

_____

_____

_____

_____

What steps are you willing to take to make sure your medical directives are honored when the time comes?

_____

_____

_____

_____

Part III

10

Our Living Spaces

"These next years are going to be about creating a life, and a living space that serves me and reflects my true nature."

—Joyce Jones, 63

The creation of an authentic living space is a process of self-discovery and one that deepens over time. Many of us spent previous years investing in and making a home for our families—living room furniture coated in Teflon, indestructible, dirt-resistant Berber carpets, bedroom dressers from garage sales, and playrooms decorated in pink Barbie furniture. Family or not, we may have spent half our lives in surroundings that didn't quite reflect our true nature. We sought a dwelling where stability and contentment were attained once and for all. Then almost as soon as that goal was achieved, a fresh desire arose—a craving for a simpler, safer, and more beautiful life.

As we age, some changes are inevitable in the environment in which we live. The homes that served us well may now be too expensive, and too difficult to keep up. We begin to explore ways to make aging more comfortable, where to live, how to avoid the danger of becoming dependent on family and children.

Some of us will resist leaving our homes and communities and choose to age in place. This choice doesn't work for all of us. Aging in place will make sense to some of us, especially if we can learn how to accept support from friends and neighbors. Many women resist asking for help when they need to be driven to the doctor or need help getting to the grocery store. This requires a level of trust and support that many independent women have never experienced.

I talked with quite a few older women before I wrote this section. Aging in their own home was a goal for a number of the independent types. Others told me they couldn't wait to get out from under the responsibility of a home that was too large or a deteriorating community. Some women told me they were ready to move and their husbands weren't; others had no vision of when or where they would go.

On some days, aging in place resonates with me—then winter comes and my sidewalks and stairs become ski slopes, and the ice builds up on my driveway and in my gutters, and in my bones; and the dreary, sunless days grab at my throat. It's inevitable—like many older people who are leaving a home where they raised their children, tended the garden, repaired the screens, and redecorated the bathroom, I will leave with a heavy heart. To save myself from jumping off my back deck and ending it all, I think positive thoughts like how liberating it will be to clean out and throw out the accumulation of stuff in my basement and attic. I fantasize about connecting with other like-minded folks and building new friendships, living new adventures in new places.

This section deals with not only where we live, but how. Some of the issues address the empty nest; organization and clutter; feng shui to reduce stress; preparing to move to a smaller, manageable home; gardening; managing on your own; retirement living; selling your house; simplifying your life; and alternatives such as shared housing, assisted living facilities, and continuing care retirement communities.

Hopefully, this section will assist you in exploring your feelings and acquiring knowledge that will enable you to make the choices you will need to make as you age.

Thoughts on Aunt Grace

"You may be wondering what Buddhism has to do with growing older, but if you can accept that 'non-attachment' is helpful, you will discover that possessions aren't as important as they were."

—Rebecca Latimer, *You're Not Old until You're Ninety*

My husband's Aunt Grace was someone I admired for who she was and how she lived her life. She was widowed for some time and living alone at 90, and we often visited her in her small, tastefully appointed one-bedroom apartment in the upscale neighborhood of Central Park West in Manhattan, New York. On one of our visits, I noticed something important about her lifestyle. She had enough money to buy out Saks Fifth Avenue, yet when she opened her closet door to retrieve her coat for a walk with us to the grocery store, I noticed only these few items:

- an umbrella
- a raincoat
- a lightweight coat for spring
- a heavy woolen coat for winter
- one pair of sturdy, fashionable overshoes
- one silk scarf and one woolen scarf
- one pair of well-made leather gloves

That was all. And this was a woman who could afford to fill her closets three times over! I never asked her why she didn't have an accumulation of things, but if I had, I'm sure she would have responded that living in a simple, uncluttered apartment made life much easier and more manageable.

Aunt Grace had a small, simple kitchen with no fancy appliances—just the basics. She and several of her older neighbors checked in on each other daily. Grace loved being around people and around culture and the arts, so Manhattan suited her. No retirement home for her! In fact, she lived happily on her own, in her apartment until she died in her mid-nineties.

Use the space below to write about an older woman whose lifestyle you admire:

_____

_____

_____

_____

_____

_____

_____

_____

_____

Staying in Your Home

"The people who are flourishing today are people who are planning for 40 or 50 more years of life after they hit midlife."

—Gail Sheehy, *New Passages*

Despite our hopes of staying in our homes forever, many of us are without the necessary amenities. If we're going to manage to do this, we have to be realistic.

You will need to consider what architectural features will make your house elder-friendly, as well as those community characteristics and services that will help you continue to live in your home as you age.

Some of the changes and modifications you will need to consider include installing grab bars in bathrooms, levers (instead of doorknobs), nonslip flooring, an emergency alert system, wide doorways, and entrances without steps. A bedroom and full bath on the main level make it easier for you to live on one floor. A safe neighborhood is important, and so is living near a hospital or other healthcare facility, with a grocery or drugstore nearby.

The community should offer transportation, preferably door-to-door, home-delivered meals, and services that offer to do errands and chores. There appears to be some denial among those who are aging. We focus on our needs for the next five years or so, but neglect what we'll need later in life. Take care of identifying and installing some of what you need now to stay in your home in the future, then sit back and relax and enjoy your life.

My inspiration for aging in place is Aunt Grace, whom we met a few pages ago. With a few modest arrangements, she stayed in her Manhattan apartment until she died at 95. She had a doorman to carry heavy groceries and packages, someone to clean once in a while, a few neighborhood children to run errands, and meals prepared by someone or delivered.

Another way to stay in your house is multigenerational living. There are countless numbers of younger women who need housing who would gratefully live alongside you in your own home. Some may provide you with cleaning help, companionship, and transportation in exchange for a place to live. Think about it.

How do you feel about this?

_____

_____

_____

_____

If you want to stay in your home for the rest of your life, what steps can you take now to make that a reality?

_____

_____

_____

_____

Gardening and Growing

> *"The garden is growth and change and that means loss as well as constant new treasures to make up for a few disasters."*
>
> —May Sarton, *Journal of a Solitude*

I am, I imagine, a farmer at heart. At the very least I am a gardener. Today, after weeding the garden and picking tomatoes, I washed the earthworm-scented soil from my hands and reverently placed the ripened tomatoes, over-sized zucchini, and herbs in the sink to be washed. I love the smell of fresh herbs and vegetables simmering in olive oil and garlic on a fall evening. This is the reward for hard work and a tortured back.

Just when I thought there would inevitably come a time when I'll have to limit my "farming" activities, I found three articles that inspired me to keep on digging. One of them described an 81-year-old woman who had been gardening for 60 years who keeps in shape by going to the YWCA five times a week so she can keep up with her garden. She has a healthy attitude and believes that you can't expect to keep everything perfect. She suggests that you let some wildflowers grow, relax, and enjoy the weeds. Fran Dalton, 71, grows giant pumpkins (800-plus pounds) in her secret hideaway garden plot in Newburyport, Massachusetts. She uses a special compost mixture (shredded leaves, animal hair, seaweed, manure, and rotten apples) which she hauls to her plot and tills by hand. A 2001 news article reported that Frieda Foretsch, 90, is the greenhouse manager for Holiday World in Santa Clara, Indiana.

Researchers tell us that gardening can help women 50 and over build stronger bones and that working in the garden for one hour a week is almost as effective for building bone strength as weight lifting. Of course, you should begin gradually and get a bone density test to see how much you can do without risking injury. If your doctor advises against doing strenuous gardening, consider growing and nurturing houseplants as an alternative.

If you don't have space for an outdoor garden (or don't want one) here are a few suggestions.

- Inside your house or apartment, create mini-gardens with plants, water, and rocks.
- By a window, place a bowl of water or a small fountain and surround it with houseplants.
- If space is limited, "force" the bulbs of paper-whites, tulips, daffodils, hyacinths, or crocuses in bowls filled with gravel or small stones.
- Light an aroma candle that spreads the fragrance of fresh flowers.
- Make the wall of a room a garden by hanging prints of flowering plants, birds, or paradise gardens.
- Place a bird feeder outside your window.

Gardening offers many benefits. As you plant and nurture a garden, you nurture your mind, body, and spirit as well. Gardening can also reduce stress and help control anxiety. Turning the soil, breathing fresh air, setting plants in the ground, then tending the plants as they grow will help you stay fit and healthy because gardening requires you to use all the major muscle groups. It frees the mind and connects you with spirit. If you don't have your own garden, consider starting or becoming part of a community garden, or volunteer to help a friend with theirs.

How do you feel about this?

_____

_____

_____

_____

What can you do to connect with the Earth and with growing things?

_____

_____

_____

_____

Color Your World (Feng Shui)

"No matter our decorating style—realized or aspired to—the essential spiritual grace our homes should possess is the solace of comfort."

—Sarah Ban Breathnach, *Simple Abundance*

If you have to downsize and move to a smaller place or a retirement community, this could be the perfect opportunity to consider how the placement of your furniture and the colors in your environment play a part in your living space and your life energy. Also, the chaotic environmental energies we were able to deal with when we were younger may not be suited to us now.

Consider the principles of feng shui. Beverly Audet, a feng shui practitioner in Los Angeles, says, "Feng Shui is the Chinese word for geomancy—the Art of Placement. This 3,000-year-old system analyzes and corrects the flow of energy, the life force or chi, within a home or office." She says that allowing ourselves to have personal space is a creative expression, and that the energy blockages in our homes affect our lives, our futures, and our health. Conscious awareness regarding our personal space is extremely important, especially as we age. We need all the positive energy we can muster.

Your home, big or small, can be decorated with beautiful, well-chosen pictures and lush plants, all expressing a clean, uncluttered simplicity. Harmonizing a home according to feng shui principles makes us feel welcome when we come home and gives us the opportunity to remember who we are.

Here are some examples of how feng shui affects an environment. Obstacles in our pathway affect our comings and goings in life. If a door doesn't open fully, feng shui says we're not opening to the fullness of the room. Dripping faucets leak out energy, affecting our finances because water represents wealth. Windows are the eyes of the home, so not seeing out is an obstacle to energy flow because we are unable to see the world. Healthy plants can help raise the life force within the home.

According to the principles of feng shui, color reflects emotional energy and can help us get what we want from our surroundings. It can mirror feelings or free them. For example, pink in the bedroom is for nurturing, with a touch of red somewhere to bring out your warmth and put some passion into your life. Green is the color of strength and new growth.

You can improve the quality of your life by becoming aware of the subtle influences in the environment. The environment becomes a metaphor for the circumstances of our lives. If our house is a mess, so might be the quality of our thinking, or the condition of our relationships. Whether you believe in the principles of feng shui or not, what surrounds us in our environments clearly influences our deepest psychological state.

How do you feel about this?

_____

_____

_____

_____

In what ways can you use some of the principles of feng shui in your current environment?

_____

_____

_____

_____

Soulful Living Space

"I realized that whenever we're inordinately dismal or fearful about aging, it means we've neglected life's spiritual dimension."

—Marsha Sinetar, *Don't Call Me Old—I'm Just Awakening!*

Surrounded by technological comforts, many women long for a way of life that encourages enrichment and meaning. At this time in your life in particular, you may be searching for inspiration and a sense of sacredness that is natural, practical, personal, and immediate. Something as simple as the sound of water gurgling in the bathtub, sunlight spilling on the windowsill, flowers scenting the air, and numerous other experiences invite soul to enter the rooms of our houses and apartments.

These next years in your life are meant to be soul-filled years, and it is difficult to feel connected to your soul in an environment that doesn't support you in that growth.

What feeling are you looking for in your house or apartment? Architects and builders may ask about your requirements for kitchen appliances, closet space, and other physical necessities but will seldom inquire about the qualities of soul you would like expressed in the design.

Soulful living is tied to life's particular moments like good food, meaningful conversation, genuine friends, and experiences that touch the heart. Our homes provide the setting for those moments that warm a deep place in us. A home for the soul is not the result of a particular style or design—the primary ingredient in creating a home for the soul is our conscious attention.

Creating space that supports our need to be in solitude is also important. Solitude allows us to touch the soul. If possible, create a space for meditation, prayer, study, writing, drawing, and playing music, a place where the mind and body can settle into the luminous silence of our true nature. Creating a setting in order to let go of demands and obligations gives us space to regain our center and be replenished by our inner resources.

How do you feel about this?

_____

_____

What steps can you take to make your home into a more soulful living space?

_____

_____

_____

_____

Simplifying

"Look at the things you have around your home. Do you get pleasure, or use, from all of them? Anything that doesn't qualify as either pleasurable or useful doesn't deserve house room."

—Joan Cleveland, *Simplifying Life as a Senior Citizen*

We are clearly an "overstuffed" society. How many times have you been seduced into buying one more appliance to make your life easier, one more gadget that promises to save time—one more trinket to adorn your wrist or fingers, one more garage sale item to clutter your coffee table? The list of consumer items is long and endless. My grandmother used to say, "Why give the money to the stores? Keep it for yourself." I've been thinking a lot about that lately.

One of the results of aging has been that my life has become a lot simpler. It feels like I've finally gotten life down to its essence. The superfluous has been stripped away and it's a relief to see it go. I've more to get rid of. It takes work to simplify and once it's done it feels wonderful. There is no way you can hold on to everything as you get older. Truth is, you just don't have the physical and emotional stamina. Most of all, I don't want to leave a lot of things for other people to take care of.

The biggest step you can take in simplifying your life is to own fewer objects. There's a natural tendency to believe that possessing more things will make us happy. But the things we own also take energy and resources—in a sense, they own us. Money must be spent buying and maintaining them; care and effort must be expended tending them. Take an inventory of all your possessions. Identify those that add value to your life and give you pleasure and those that don't. Consider getting rid of those possessions that cost more in time, trouble, dusting, or money to maintain than they are worth. Throwing them in the trash is an option, but I prefer recycling them: sell them in a yard sale, auction them on the Internet, give them to family and friends, or donate them to charity. Ah, freedom!

How do you feel about this?

_____

_____

_____

_____

What steps can you take today to simplify your life?

_____

_____

_____

_____

Paint and Wallpaper

"Several years ago . . . I announced that I was too old ever to hang wallpaper again, and if things got too shabby we'd have to bring in a professional."

—Madeleine L'Engle, *The Irrational Season*

When I was in my energetic early thirties, I did much of the work on my then well-worn 1928 home by myself. Climbing up and down ladders, I painted inside and out, I hung wallpaper (badly), laid flooring, refinished and assembled furniture. Now just looking at the ladder and work gloves in the basement makes me want to take a nap.

I'm still living in that dear old house, and some of the work I did 20 years ago now needs to be done again. Refinished wooden floors lose their shine; bathroom tiles turn dull; and greenish, dated wallpaper saddens a room. These things get me down and steal my energy if I let them go too long.

Like me, you may not have the strength to climb a ladder or paint a room, but what does it take to arrange a vase of flowers? How much energy does it take to pick up the phone and ask someone to paint a room for you? Sometimes all a room needs is a little spiffing up with soap and water. If you've always maintained and nurtured your home in the past as I have, it may be hard to let go and let someone else do the necessary upkeep these days.

Remember, you don't have to do it yourself. I find it a lot safer and a great deal more entertaining to sit and watch others do it for me these days, or to leave the house and come back to find it done!

How do you feel about this?

_____

_____

_____

_____

Make a list of friends, family, or professionals you can trust who might be willing to help you make your living environment clean, safe, and attractive.

_____

_____

_____

_____

_____

_____

_____

_____

Selling Your House

"If we are still trying to figure out how to care for our too large house and garden, and what to do with all our goods and chattels, we can't let go into a new life."

—Marion Woodman, in *On Women Turning 60* by Cathleen Rountree

In preparation for a future time, I am cleaning, sorting, and throwing away things today. As my husband and I age, and/or I am widowed, someday the house I live in will need to be sold. Perhaps you're thinking about it, too. So I'm downsizing now—simplifying—while I still have lots of energy and a solid mind for organizing.

If you are thinking about selling your home because either you or your partner are disabled, remember there are affordable nonmedical services for people who prefer to remain at home, where their quality of life is enhanced without the stress and hardships of interrupted routines and changes in daily habits. These services are designed for people capable of managing their physical needs, but who require limited assistance, light housework, and/or companionship in order to remain at home.

Even if you live in a rental, co-op, or condo, sometime in the future you may have to move to a place where there aren't as many steps or rooms to keep up, or where there are facilities or relatives nearby in case you need them—where the cost of living is easier on your budget, where you can walk to the supermarket, where there are people your own age.

If you do need to sell your home, there are some simple things you can do to make your home more appealing and to help sell it a bit faster:

- Out front—look at your house from the street. If you need to, get someone to help you trim the hedges and bushes. Then add a coat of semigloss paint to the front door and buy a brand new doormat. Polish the doorknob. Out back—clean up the patio and deck. Repair or get rid of broken, discolored outdoor furniture.

- Unclutter the entryway and hang a mirror. Mirrors can help any room look more spacious. Consider putting a vase of flowers on an entryway table to greet potential buyers.

- In the dining room—consider removing the leaves from your dining room table to make the room look bigger. In the kitchen—take down the refrigerator magnets and the grandkids' drawings from the refrigerator door, and put away the large countertop appliances.

In general, get rid of as much clutter as possible before putting your house on the market. An uncluttered house looks larger and more attractive to buyers. Clear out everything you no longer use or don't expect to need when you move.

How do you feel about this?

_____

_____

_____

_____

List a few things you can start doing now to make your home more desirable and easier to sell when the time comes:

_____

_____

_____

_____

Retirement Living Spaces

"We can't rely on others to plan our retirement, because each of us has our own unique realm where we want to be."

—Marion E. Haynes, *Comfort Zones*

We all seek a level of comfort in our lives. Among other things, we desire living where we want to live, doing things we enjoy doing, and creating work in the world that brings us a sense of satisfaction. To retire successfully, one needs to strive for staying within a defined comfort zone while making the transition from full time work.

It may seem too soon to consider where to live in retirement, especially when you are strong and healthy, energetic, and living comfortably in a community where you have good support services, friends, and family. However, this is a very good time to investigate possible future living arrangements. You don't want to delay the search until you are sick or injured, or have lost a husband who could have been helpful in the decision-making process. Take your time, and the search may even end up being enjoyable.

If you are like most women contemplating retirement and relocation, the factors that will most likely affect your future quality of life are where the children and grandchildren are living, housing, climate, economics, healthcare, personal safety, and access to recreational and cultural activities. These days you can do a lot of your search online. I read about something called the Retirement Living Information Center (www.retirementliving.com), where you can choose from one of six types of facilities and then search by city and state. You can get information about the nearest city, the weather there, maps, and other details.

As far as I'm concerned, I think it's better to take a long, hard look into the future and not be caught off guard. Of course, life is unpredictable—I'm not denying that. But I want to be a participant in the process of life and have some say in where I spend my days.

How do you feel about this?

_____

_____

_____

_____

Where do you see yourself living in retirement? Where would you feel most "at home"?

_____

_____

_____

_____

Downsizing: Preparing a Move
to a Smaller, More Manageable Home

"Ten years ago I decided to simplify my life. I got rid of roomfuls of possessions and moved from a big house to a condominium. I have never missed anything I gave away . . . and I have felt much lighter of heart and mind since."

—Elaine St. James, *Simplify Your Life*

Many of us feel the need to downsize and simplify as time moves on. It's part of life's process. It may be time to consider moving to a smaller, more manageable house or to an apartment or condo, or assisted living—to someplace that better suits your needs. Maybe you've been banging around in a large, overwhelming, outdated house for just too long and you're good and ready to make the change. Others of you may be content just where you are for the time being. It may feel uncomfortable to think about, but as we age, creating a manageable living environment is a necessity.

I find myself worrying from time to time about how I'll make the transition. Will I be able to create the kind of nurturing nest I know I'll require for my sunset years, a place that will support my body, mind, and spirit? Louise L. Hay wrote an inspiring affirmation in her book, *Heal Your Body:* "I provide myself a comfortable home, one that fills all my needs and is a pleasure to be in. I fill the rooms with the vibration of love so that all who enter, myself included, will feel the love and be nourished by it."

I think that's where I'll start. When the time comes, I'll fill my new home with the vibration of love, and let it happen from there. I know there are lots of things that I will gladly let go of, the kind of material stuff that depletes my life force. In *Journey to the Heart*, Melody Beattie tells us: "Objects have energy, they have energy in them when we obtain them, and they have the energy and meaning we attribute to them. Choose carefully the possessions you want around you, for they tell a story all day long."

So, begin to think about downsizing. Make a conscious effort not to buy stuff you will later have to make space for in a smaller home, or stuff you will have to get rid of when the time comes. The act of letting go of the burden of caring for too many possessions will leave more room to fill your home with the vibration of love.

How do you feel about this?

_____

_____

_____

_____

If you decide to move to a smaller, more manageable home someday, how would you like it to look?

_____

_____

_____

_____

What can you do now to prepare for this transition?

_____

_____

_____

_____

Living Alone and Liking It

"When I am an old, old woman I may very well be living all alone like many another before me."

—Kate Barnes, "Future Plans," in *Where the Deer Were*

Statistics indicate that 36 percent of women over age 65 live alone and that about 45 percent of the total population of older Americans are single. Chances are you may find yourself living alone one day and wondering how to make the best of it.

Two of my favorite authors have positive thoughts on the topic of living alone. Frances Weaver says, "Living alone means I can eat all of the Pepperidge Farm cookies without feeling I must hide the empty sack." Carolyn. G. Heilbrun writes, "The solitude of old age is often pleasurable, offering, I sometimes think, a pleasure similar to those described by converts to a religion." I agree.

On the other hand, if I don't want to live alone, what alternatives do I have? I consider what it would be like to live with my children, or to live around or in the company of younger people. Intergenerational living has its drawbacks. The difficulties arise from trying to combine what is essentially two different cultures. It feels like it would be a matter of disparate tempos. The younger generation can feel like they're moving nonstop in all they do, and they will probably find that we move too slowly. Our patience may become exhausted and it doesn't matter how much we love and care for each other.

A very wise person once said, "The old are younger in each other's presence." We need to be with others like us, others who understand our unreliable memories and our need for routine. Of course, it can be refreshing to visit with our younger family members, children, and friends. But, admit it—isn't it a relief when they leave? Barbara Holland said in *One's Company*, "No doubt about it, solitude is improved by being voluntary. . . . If you live with other people, their temporary absence can be refreshing." So I entertain the idea of living alone in my later years. Of course, it would be great to have my husband with me, and I have to be prepared because that may not happen.

My sister, Marilyn, who lived alone for many years, came up with some innovative ways to care for yourself when you live alone:

1. Have the newspaper delivered daily. The regularity of that event each morning can make you mindful of the things in life you can count on.

2. If you don't already have one, get an electric coffeepot with a timer. Set it the night before, and wake to the scent of coffee or tea as a welcoming way to start your day. You can do the same with a programmable bread maker.

3. During good weather, plan in advance to have a neighborhood youngster shovel snow for you in winter, or weed for you in the summer. Make a snack for them during a break and have a chat.

The Next Fifty Years

4. Install night lights in every room of the house. Especially useful are the ones that come on automatically as the house dims. Coming home to a dark house and getting up in the night to a dark house can be unpleasant when one lives alone. Or if you prefer, put up small white Christmas lights on a fake ficus tree or a wicker bookcase. It's amazing how comforting they are.

5. Buy yourself flowers—some beautiful bundles are less than five dollars at the grocery store.

6. Burn incense—the scent will enhance your feelings of well-being and relaxation.

7. Play beautiful music and soak in a hot bathtub with bubbles up to your chin.

8. Plug in a small TV in the kitchen. It's good company.

9. Adopt a pet from the shelter—it will love you unconditionally. If you're allergic to pets, buy yourself a stuffed animal.

10. Buy a portable "heat dish" to warm your damp or winter days. You can take it from room to room with you. You'll feel cozy and save money on utilities.

11. Subscribe to an Internet service provider and e-mail friends and family.

12. Replace your old scratchy polyester blend sheets with soft cotton or flannel, and wash them and toss them in the dryer with a great-smelling fabric softener. Invest in a down comforter or feather bed (like sleeping on a cloud in the arms of love), and buy yourself the coziest pajamas and slippers you can find.

13. Invite a friend to your house for lunch or dinner at least once a week.

14. Keep a list of positive affirmations about yourself in a prominent place, and read it daily.

15. When you're out in the world, smile a lot, and people will smile back at you.

Living alone is an opportunity to get to know yourself better, to get in touch with your inner resources, and living alone is a choice, not a sentence. How do you feel about this?

_____

_____

_____

_____

If you live alone now, or plan to in the future, how would you like your environment to be?

_____

_____

_____

_____

Empty Nests with Silver Linings

"I've reached the stage where I'm no longer able to call myself middle-aged because that's what my children are."

—Judith Viorst, *Suddenly Sixty*

I'm on my way to 60, and it's taken about five years to become totally comfortable with the fact that my children are doing well on their own and my nest is empty. For some of you, the nest is empty because you were care-giving one or both of your parents who are no longer living with you. Or you are now living without your spouse.

This is an opportunity to create a space that is uniquely your own. One room to call your very own. One corner of the apartment reclaimed. One whole house to design any way you wish. Not only can you redesign your environment, but you can eat what and when you'd like, walk around naked after your shower, and surf the TV channels whenever you're in the mood. You can

The Next Fifty Years

fill your home with friends who like to drink martinis; you can play your music loud.

How do you feel about this?

_____

_____

_____

_____

When, and if, the time comes that your nest is empty, what do you imagine doing in and with the newly acquired space?

_____

_____

_____

_____

_____

_____

_____

Clutter: You Can't Take It with You!

"A regular, serious attack on mess and unnecessary clutter, performed with a glad heart, makes you feel in control of all the parts of your life you care about."

—Alexandra Stoddard, *Living a Beautiful Life*

Are you at risk for burial under an avalanche of stuff each time you open a closet door? A wise someone once said that we spend the first half of our lives collecting and buying stuff and the second half of our lives trying to get rid of it all! Mary C. Morrison once remarked that although our houses may be empty of people, they are still full of an accumulation of things, and "our lives are encrusted with possessions and burdened with the work they entail."

Lately I've been asking myself if I want my children to have to row through a sea of clutter when I'm gone. I imagine the burden it would create for them. "Who wants Mom's drawerfull of candle stubs?" (I've been meaning to melt them down to make new candles.) "Who wants Mom's vintage 1970s blouses?" (I've been hoping they would come back in style.) "Who wants Mom's stained linen napkins?" (I've been waiting until I had enough of them to put in a dark dye bath to hide the stains.) You may not have children, but consider the fact that your partner, other family members, or friends will eventually have to deal with your stuff.

My goal each day is to find one thing to donate, throw out, or give away. It's amazing how many things I've been holding on to that are no longer of use. When we're ready to get real about our clutter, organizing gurus tell us that we should create three bags or boxes that say, "Garbage," "Give Away," and "Put Someplace Else," and a fourth that says "Undecidable." They suggest visiting your "undecidable" box after a few weeks and toss or give away anything you haven't retrieved in that time. My system is to keep a shopping bag behind my bedroom door and the minute I have the thought, "Why am I holding on to this?" into the Goodwill bag it goes.

How do you feel about this?

_____

_____

_____

_____

Have you been holding on to too much stuff? Like what?

_____

_____

_____

_____

What steps can you take today to begin the process of letting go and lightening up?

_____

_____

_____

_____

Leaving Home

"At 67, I'm selfish enough to want my own way. I want to be with my own generation, people who understand the issues I live with. . . . Living with my children would have been a burden on me and on them. So I live in a home with lots of people my age."

—"Bertha," 67, from *You Are Not Alone*

It's a quiet Sunday afternoon. As I look out at the familiar views from each window of the house I've lived in for the last 23 years, I wonder how much I'll miss it when I need to move from here one day. Some days I imagine I'll shoot a photograph out each of the windows and assemble the pictures into an album that I can take with me. Other days I know that the next step in my evolution will need to be taken with courage, no looking back, no photographs to remind me of what I've left.

I remember some of the older women I've met along the way who were devastated when they had to leave their homes and go into an assisted living or long-term residential care facility. A series of upheavals had brought them to this part of the journey—their health was uncertain, they had lost their economic independence, and they usually had no options for ever leaving the institution—they typically felt vulnerable and frightened on every level. Although it may seem the right thing to do at the right time for all involved, the decision to move into a new life pattern will undoubtedly be a hard time for me—for all of us. It becomes a time when we must leave the familiar setting and a past we have lived with and loved.

Perhaps I will consider sharing my home to escape the trap of retreating into an institution. We have options. In some areas there are social service programs coordinating these living arrangements. But if I do have to leave, I've made a pledge to myself that when the time comes to live in a facility for the aging, I will prepare to leave my home in gentle stages.

Author Mary C. Morrison describes moving from one's home as "a real wrench" that "brings another of the gifts of old age, the chance to say goodbye—a long, deep, fully conscious farewell." I will slowly and carefully give away my possessions as the time approaches. I will say goodbye to the familiar. I will do a leave-taking ceremony where I go through my home room by room, saying goodbye to each room; perhaps I'll say a prayer or remove a small memento from each room as I go. It doesn't have to be sad. It's so much better to grieve the loss and get on with it than not have the time to say goodbye.

I will not plunge into a serious depression or become anxious. I tell myself that these days there are many resources for providing retirement community residents with wonderful opportunities for art, exercise, community work, and socializing, in addition to good medical care. Some facilities even offer field trips, fitness instructors, dancing, painting and cooking classes, gardening, and bridge. I cheer myself with the fact that in the 1950s the average age of persons entering nursing homes was 65, while now the age of admission is closer to 85. So you and I have some time to plan and get used to the idea.

How do you feel about this?

_____

_____

_____

_____

What will you do to make the transition easier for yourself when the time comes?

_____

_____

_____

_____

11

Our Families

"I'm beginning to think about what it will be like to be 70-80-90 and I see myself surrounded by friends and family as I have been my whole life."

—Patty Thomma, 60

As we age, our families become helpful and supportive, or neglectful and critical—they either value us or don't. How they treat us is often a reflection of how we see ourselves. If we don't see ourselves as worthwhile contributors to society and approach our aging with dignity and respect for ourselves, how can we expect them to see us that way?

I had lunch with my 32-year-old daughter the other day, and she spent half the time talking about how society needs to readjust its attitudes towards its aging population. She reassured me that I would always be a valuable person in her life and that she would care for me, no questions asked, when I was older. I was grateful for her affirmation of our relationship and, at the same time, concerned that I would ever become a burden to her and her family. She reminded me that my attitude needed "an adjustment," that I shouldn't see myself as becoming a burden to her or anyone else.

While I was writing this, my husband called from his office to say that his son (from a previous marriage), Jacob, had just been hospitalized because of concerns about his heart. Between us we have five grown children—my husband has two and I have three. His call caused me to evaluate our role in the parenting of older children, and I'm thinking how important our families are to us. How much we rely on each other for guidance, support, and security. How, as we age, our children are aging with us.

Our greater longevity has brought fundamental changes to our lives of which we are hardly aware or that we take for granted. Experts tell us that in 1920, for example, ten-year-olds in the United States had only a 40 percent chance of having two of their possible four grandparents alive. But these days that figure is 80 percent.

This section addresses such issues as how we relate to our families, creating a family history, and the joys and challenges of grandmothering. It also discusses shared holidays, special events, and general family issues such as our changing roles and expectations within the family as we age, dealing with grown children, caring for aging relatives, and what we can expect from our sons and daughters as we age.

An Easy-to-Visit Elder

I've decided to be an easy-to-visit elder
    to consider my effect on those
    who come by to see me
    to engage in their lives and mine
I'll plan for them to need me
    and not have a desperate need for them
I will not put my Ancient Mariner
    stranglehold on them
    with my tales of tiresome sorrows
Instead we'll exchange wisdom for energy
Exchange a story for some news
Eat home-made cakes
Drink fresh ground coffee
I want to be loved by younger people
    to have an open heart
    an easy laugh
    an infectious appreciation of every moment
I will douse my fiery moral judgments
with the water of enthusiasm and wisdom
I will offer them a haven filled with peace
and perspective,
    ask what they think and
    really listen

—P. D. Blair

Many of the younger generation complain that their elders (relatives or not) are tedious to visit. Perhaps we are because we haven't considered our effect on their visit with us. We bore them because we haven't kept up with the times, or we're too focused on our physical ailments. By the time we're 65 or so, most of us have at least five chronic conditions and nobody wants to hear about them, especially in detail.

In *Let Evening Come: Reflections on Aging*, Mary C. Morrison tells us "chances to enjoy the beauty of youth depend greatly upon whether or not the young enjoy being with us." If they enjoy being with us, all we really have to do is be there for them and they will visit as often as they can. She reminds us to be an elder that feels at home with themselves and in touch with what is going on in the world.

How do you feel about this?

_____

_____

_____

_____

Think back to when you were younger and describe an older woman you enjoyed visiting and what made it special.

_____

_____

_____

_____

Moving to the Circumference

"I personally prefer to speak of this stage of adult development as a journey, a movement toward a new, unknown destination."

—Joyce Rupp

Imagine life as a series of circles, growing wider and wider, spinning us to the outer edge where eventually life feels satisfying and you become willing to pass the baton to the next generation. At this stage it may feel right and good to step down as family leader and decision-maker. The younger generation can now be free to make their own decisions. They can handle their own family's affairs just as you did for your family for many years.

The holidays are a time when you may sense that movement toward the circumference, where we are still part of the family circle but are no longer in the center. Take Thanksgiving, for example. I envision a day in the not too distant future when my house will no longer be the destination for everyone on that day. There's a part of me that resists that inevitability, and a part of me that is more than willing to give up the job of basting the turkey all day.

Mary C. Morrison in *Let Evening Come* refers to this time of life as "a marvelous, warm place" that "waits for us on the periphery of family life; all it asks of us is to live along gently into it, aware of its promises and possibilities."

Let's face it, we've spent the best years of our lives learning multitasking, the complicated managerial skills that family life requires, to a point where they have become second nature to us. How can we possibly let them go? Sooner or later we must do so, and the goal is to do so as gracefully as possible.

How do you feel about this?

_____

_____

_____

_____

Imagine you are at the circumference. Describe what a holiday or other family gathering would look like from that new perspective:

_____

_____

_____

_____

_____

_____

_____

_____

New Grandma

"We look in those little faces and see a miraculous blending of generations and genes: a grandfather's cheekbones, a mother's eyes, a sibling's dimples. And that fresh new face composed of familiar parts reminds us of loved ones living and gone and of all the emotions and history we've shared with them."

—Barbara Johnson, *Living Somewhere between Estrogen and Death*

To fully experience the special event of your first grandchild, you might want to plan to be there for the delivery if you can. Find out the hospital rules from the doctor who'll be performing the delivery. Sometimes grandparents are allowed in the delivery room, especially if it's their own daughter, perhaps in the background to respect the mother's modesty. Helping my daughter, Aimee, give birth was an incredible experience. If you can't witness the birth, you can be in the waiting room. Then you can hold the newborn and present your new grandchild with her first teddy bear. Not only should you be there to welcome the new baby, you should thank the new parents for the gift of a grandchild.

Don't be disappointed if the new parents don't want anyone—even grandparents—in the hospital at all. If that's the case, let the parents-to-be decide how to keep you posted. Coordinate your plans with those of the other grandparents to avoid any conflicts. If it's impossible to be at the birth or in the hospital while it's happening, try to make a trip to see the infant, and the parents, as soon as you can. Discuss the visit with the parents-to-be so you'll be able to comply with their wishes. A grandchild's birth can bring a distant family together, and with you on the scene to welcome the baby, the occasion can become a family celebration.

If you're adrift as to how to be helpful, appoint yourself the family reporter, recording the birth and accompanying celebration with a camera or a video camera. Ask the parents what they need. Chances are the new parents will have their hands very, very full, and your presence can be a great help to them. The new baby's siblings will need the kind of attention and support that a loving grandmother can provide so well. But remember, we grandparents, as visitors or surrogates, must learn to take our clues from the parents in order not to undermine their authority.

The new parents may not have provided anything to eat for their return home. If that's the case, why not bring in something special for the happy couple, so they'll have meals for several days? Grandparents can help in countless ways, from basic housekeeping to making sure that older grandchildren get to and from school and play dates, etc. If there's no live-in housekeeper, one grandparent may actually move in for a while to ease the burden.

How do you feel about this?

_____

_____

_____

_____

Is there anything about this experience that you are uncomfortable with? In what way could you feel most useful during this time?

_____

_____

_____

_____

Grandmothering 101
(Even if you have no grandchildren of your own)

"A grandmother is a lady who has no little children of her own. She likes other people's."

—An anonymous eight-year-old

We don't necessarily have to give birth to a child to leave a legacy. My grandmother worked as a nanny and housekeeper for several families. At her funeral, the children she cared for, now in their 50s and 60s, lined up to pay their respects to her and to tell us the kind of positive, nurturing impact she had on their lives.

Being a grandmother these days isn't easy. The role of grandparent has a way of splitting your personality into two opposing halves. One half of you believes in the traditional grandparent—the soft, warm, dependable, always-there kind you enjoyed when you were a kid. The other half is living energetically in the present, enjoying the freedoms that are finally possible.

An AARP study suggests that most grandparents play an interested, active role in their grandchildren's lives. Despite busy lives and geographic separation, grandparents over 50 enjoy a strong closeness between the generations. Some even spend time with their grandchildren every day and are regular caregivers.

Many grandparents see their role as a companion or confidante. They give advice and share stories from the good old days. When visiting they enjoy eating together, watching TV programs, shopping for clothes, playing sports, and attending church.

Grandparents have helped raise grandchildren throughout history, and many have done it full time. Today's grandmother loves her children and grandchildren, and most will do anything in the world for them, yet she refuses to follow the script for the typical grandmother and live at their beck and call.

Remember that it's not too late to be a better grandmother than you were a mother. We hear so much about old conflicts resurfacing between parents and adult children. The birth and growth of grandchildren offer tremendous possibilities for repair and enrichment between the two older generations. Your child may ask for your advice in ways he or she never did at 17. Now you have more self-knowledge than you did when you were a young parent.

Our grandchildren may look to us for unconditional love and comfort when they are younger. Staying close to grandchildren can make it possible for you to help them through difficult times as they get older. Lillian Carson in *The Essential Grandparent* reminds us to "Stay in touch when grandchildren become teenagers. They often need someone other than friends to talk to. Keep a grandchild's confidence unless you feel his parents must know." Have one-on-one time with each grandchild starting when he or she is very young. Then talk will flow naturally as he gets older. It's a privilege to give them what they can't get from anyone else. We are "parental," we are closely related, and we can give without an expectation of getting.

Here are some ideas and actions to keep in mind as you learn the grandmothering role:

- We need to learn to get along with, or cope with, the other grandparents who want time with the children also.

- Be sensitive to the values and disciplinary rules that the parents have for your grandchildren.

- Let them know that you have no desire to turn yourself into their on-call babysitter. (The irritation you feel when adult children take your time for granted can grow into seething resentment.)

- You deserve to enjoy your retirement years, guilt-free. You do not want to meddle or control the lives of your children or grandchildren.

How do you feel about this?

_____

_____

_____

_____

In what other ways would you like to be involved in the life of your grandchildren (or another small child)?

_____

_____

_____

_____

What other rules or guidelines would you like to add to the ones mentioned above?

_____

_____

_____

_____

Distance Grandparenting

"Knowing how to be a grandmother does not come instinctively, any more than knowing how to be a mother simply flows in a woman's blood. Nature may help, but basically it's a learned activity."

—Sheila Kitzinger, *Becoming a Grandmother*

My good friend Ginena Dulley Wills said, "One of my greatest pleasures in midlife and beyond continues to be my family. I have found that keeping in touch with two adult sons, daughters-in-law, and four grandsons in distant places takes energy and intentionality on the part of each of us."

I asked Ginena to contribute to this essay by offering advice to other grandmothers living a distance away from their grandkids. To my delight, she came up with this advice based on her experiences:

Mail: I am always prepared to take the initiative and am not necessarily surprised if I don't receive a response as often or as soon as I would like. I keep my letters short and simple, especially for the younger ones. They don't have the patience to listen to long letters. When on vacation or traveling, I send postcards, pictures, and brochures of where we have been. Later I often see them on the front of the fridge when I go to visit. Because one family lives in the south it is fun to send dried leaves for the grandchildren to look at. I often include a stick of gum or a fridge magnet along with the letter.

Phone: I again take the initiative and don't wait around for those phone calls. They are busy people. I try to be sensitive to the family routine so they are more likely to be available when I call, but a cheery message on the answering machine seems also to be appreciated. Younger children don't always respond while on the telephone, but they are probably smiling and nodding their heads as they enjoy listening. I try to keep abreast of what is happening in the lives of my children and grandchildren so that I can call shortly before or after an event to share their excitement.

Fax and e-mail: I enjoy keeping in touch with my grandchildren through their drawings. My son will sometimes fax something one of the boys has created (homework and A-plus essays). That way they can keep the original and I still get to see it. We frequently exchange pictures online. They can be scanned into the computer or use a digital camera. E-mail is a way of keeping in touch, with messages once or twice a week to update everyone on what is happening in our lives, or send greeting cards for special occasions—everyone likes to get mail! We sometimes schedule to be available to chat back and forth online.

Video: Video cameras have added a new dimension to keeping in touch on a frequent basis. It is great to be able to see special events as well as what they are doing in their everyday lives. We have recently moved, and this is a way to share our new neighborhood and living space with those who won't be able to come to visit very soon. I find it is so important to visit my children and grandchildren on a regular basis. Making the time to celebrate a special birthday, program at school, or special event in life is what keeps us close and connected to each other—you will never regret it.

I think Ginena's ideas are great. Now here are some of my own:

- Schedule regular telephone times. To assist your memory and to make sure you ask the questions that will make for good conversation, make a list of things you want to talk about in between chats.

- Record bedtime stories on audio or videotape, perhaps a chapter at a time. One grandmother I know videotapes herself doing puppet shows.

- Share a movie or book you enjoyed or you think they might enjoy. After you've watched it or read it, send it through the mail, then talk about it during one of your scheduled phone calls.

- Offer to babysit the children for a weekend so the parents can get away.

- Buy your grandchild a disposable camera. Have them shoot pictures of their neighborhood, school, friends, and pets, then send you the film for developing.

- Start a separate travel savings fund—to bring them to you, or you to them.

How do you feel about long-distance grandparenting?

_____

_____

_____

_____

Write down at least one way you would be willing to stay in touch with your grandchildren:

_____

_____

_____

_____

Caregiving Grandchildren

"I haven't found anything wonderful about being older . . . you start losing things—your hair, your hearing, your eyesight. What you don't want to lose is the ability to help people who need you."

—Helen Gurley Brown, at age 78

According to U.S. census figures, the number of caregiving grandparents increased by about 44 percent in the last ten years. So, more and more grandparents are being summoned back into service. Just when we thought it was time to retire, relax, travel, and watch *Oprah.*

Research shows when older people care for others, their mental health improves. Giving massages, owning pets, and being matched with surrogate grandchildren have all been shown to reduce depression and stress.

On the other hand, I came across a study in the September/October 2004 *Archives of Family Medicine* saying that too much caregiving can have the opposite effect! Like when grandparents become the primary caregivers for their grandchildren. Seems those grandparents are twice as likely to be depressed as non-caregiving grandparents. The researchers postulate that it might be the exhaustion, isolation, and financial and physical stress (especially caring for toddlers). This sounds similar to what I experienced when I was a young mother. Who didn't want to run away from home and responsibility during those exhausting years and sign themselves into a locked ward?

For a variety of reasons, some grandmothers are caring for a grandchild full time. In this case it's important to not go it alone. There are about 400 to 500 grandparent caregiver support groups around the country and respite programs so grandma can take the weekend off. Try the Grandparent Information Center of the American Association of Retired Persons (AARP) for some resources or start a support group for grandmas in your community.

If you're caregiving a grandchild, it can be an enormously rewarding experience. I loved caring for my grandson after school (when he still needed me). His 3:15 P.M. arrival offered a welcome break in my day and a chance to activate my own inner child—milk and cookies, homework help, and an occasional game of gin rummy.

How do you feel about your role as grandparent/caregiver?

_____

_____

_____

_____

If you don't have grandchildren (or ones that don't live nearby), in what ways can you can share your gifts with a younger child in your community?

_____

_____

_____

_____

Caregiving Our Parents

"In the past year, I lost my mother to cancer and helped my father move to a retirement home. I'm proud of the way I rose to the occasion. I learned that I can manage more than I thought I could!"

—Sally, 55

Women in this society are generally the hands-on caregivers, and we're very good at guilt. Guilt can become mingled with resentment and rage. We think, how much of my life am I supposed to give up to do this? If you are asking this question, perhaps the burden of care is not equally distributed among your family members. The older population continues to grow, thanks to modern medicine. In the next 50 years, women, who have become the default caregivers of our society, could end up in this role for much of their lives.

Be ready to compromise; delegate responsibilities; ask for help whenever possible; and don't neglect your own physical, emotional, and mental health. If you try to do it all, you've set yourself up for failure. Set boundaries; try to see your time together as a gift and a way of deepening your relationship. While caring for an elderly parent, we can learn many coping skills from them. If someone has made it to 80 or 90 years old, they've done something right. If you stop running around, you might learn something valuable from them. Sit down for an hour, reminisce about old times, or page through an old photo album together. If you see caregiving a parent as a burden, it will become one. On the other hand, if you see it as a challenge, you will feel rewarded and proud of yourself each time you resolve a conflict or a problem.

Here are some suggestions for managing the caregiving:

- Consult a geriatrician, a doctor who specializes in seniors and is tuned into quality-of-life issues, especially if the primary care doctor doesn't seem to be adequately addressing your parent's concerns.

- Depression is a prevalent problem among the elderly and is widely under-recognized and undertreated, so familiarize yourself with the signs.

- Know the details about what treatment your parents would want should they become unable to make decisions (i.e., living will, healthcare proxy, or healthcare power of attorney).

- If your parents want to stay in their own community, find out about the resources available there.

Now it's time for you. Make a list of actions you could take that would nourish your body, mind, and spirit. Write one action on your calendar every day, and do it. Listen to music, sit in a chapel, take a walk. Gather information on diet, exercise, and stress reduction. Confide in someone like a nonjudgmental sibling, close friend, or neighbor. Find a support group for caregivers.

If you are caregiving a parent, what actions can you take that would benefit them?

_____

_____

_____

_____

What actions can you take that would benefit you?

_____

_____

_____

_____

Parenting "Old" Children

"Denial is believing that your adult children and their spouses will appreciate your setting them straight on everything from where they should live to what they should eat."

—Judy Sheindlin ("Judge Judy"), _Keep It Simple, Stupid_

If you are 50-plus and have children, they are likely to be 20 to 30 years old. If you're 60-plus, they are 30-plus, if you're 70-plus they may be in their 40s and 50s. The question remains, what is our role as parents of our grown children and how do we "parent" and relate to these old kids? What do we do when the kids hit us up for a loan, or move back home . . . or use our homes for storage!? How do we react when they want to butt into our business?

One of my good friends said, "First of all, stay away from your 'old' children as much as possible. They not only make you look older, but they can actually make you _feel_ older." I say, if staying away from your "old" children is not possible or would be unkind, consider buying them a facelift. Well, it's not possible to stay away from them forever, so we need to learn to live among them on the same planet.

Florida Scott-Maxwell wrote in *The Measure of My Days* that "no matter how old a mother is she watches her middle-aged children for signs of improvement." This couldn't be more true for me. No only do I watch for signs of improvement in my children, I sometimes find myself wanting to live their lives so I can change their outcomes to an easier one for me to look at! As my 32-year-old single daughter Aimee reminds me, "You bother me sometimes. You worry about my relationships too much. Just listen when I talk and stop trying to fix things so I can feel free to learn and mature from my own trials and errors." In *Growing Older, Getting Better*, Jane Porcino writes that "this is a time to develop both autonomy and relatedness."

Is your urge to meddle in your adult children's lives so overwhelming that you just can't help yourself? I can't tell you how many times I've slipped back into treating my adult son and daughter like they're eight years old. "Wear your jacket, it's cold outside," or "Are you eating enough vegetables?" It's hard to let go of the mother role and to see your children as adults. To add to the difficulty, some young adults take a very long time and follow a very circuitous route before they eventually find their way in the world.

These days, close to 20 million young adults live with their parents, and that doesn't count all those who boomeranged back more than once. Jean, 59, told me, "I waved goodbye to my youngest offspring, squaring my shoulders and gritting my teeth as I turned to do battle with the empty nest demons. Three months later he was back!" A goodly percentage of "kids" 25 to 34 are still living in their family homes, and some never left. Some "boomerang kids" (young adults over 18 returning to the family nest) may rotate in and out for years, if not decades, changing the household's dynamics, sometimes for the better, sometimes for the worse. Financial pressures are most likely to send adult children back to the nest.

If your son or daughter shows up on your doorstep, you will need a clear plan. The plan should cover rent and other financial contributions, chores, house rules about such things as visitors and smoking, and any other expectations you have. Keep a united front with your spouse so your child doesn't pit one of you against the other. Set a limit on how long they can stay. Encourage your child to move on with his life and to create a well-defined plan. Adult children still crave our approval, and we must not judge their behavior in the same way we did when they were young. Our corrections and suggestions can have a negative emotional impact. When parents and adult children live far apart, their brief visits can turn into replays of child/parent relationships that might turn explosive.

By all means, don't ignore the obvious. If the child has a drug problem, deal with it right away. Any kindness you offer should be conditional upon his enrollment in a treatment program. Otherwise, you are enabling him.

Our kids aren't kids anymore. They're over 21 and they're supposed to behave like adults, and when they don't it's hard to hold your tongue. As a wise friend once told me, when you get to that age in your life when your children have husbands or wives and you see things your children or your sons-in-law or daughters-in-law are doing that you don't approve of, keep it to yourself—even if you think it was your faulty parenting that created the hardship.

If you're a parent, you know that guilt is a constant companion. It's not surprising that a generation like ours, which prides itself on self-reflection, ends up blaming itself for our children's failure to thrive in the world. It's crucial that we stop thinking like that. The key to our sanity and survival, as well as theirs, is detachment—not from our children, but from their problems. We must acknowledge the limits of our parental responsibility and accept that we have done as much as we possibly could for them.

How do you feel about this?

_____

_____

_____

_____

How can you continue to be a part of your children's lives in a healthy, balanced way?

_____

_____

_____

_____

Changing Places: Moving in with Your Kids

"Inside every older person there's a younger person wondering what happened."

—Ashleigh Brilliant, from the Internet

So many uncomfortable emotions click into place when I consider living with my children someday in the future. The only thought that comes to mind on this topic is, "payback is a bitch." I could move in with my adult kids some day and act like a teenager—that would teach them a lesson, wouldn't it?

But on a serious note, I feel that most of us put this option at the bottom of the list of choices for living out our old age. I can imagine that for some of you it would be a joy to be around grandchildren, to feel useful in some way, to be part of a family once again. In some cultures, it is mandatory to care for one's parents at home. Since I like some measure of control over my environment and a lot of peace and quiet, it would make me miserable unless I had a completely separate apartment connected to their house, or a small bungalow on their property.

My daughter has already announced that she will never put me in a nursing home to be neglected or abused, as she puts it. If I am ill and need care, I see moving in with her and her family as one big pain in the ass for all of them and me as well. Do I want to end my life being a pain in the ass to someone?

M. F. K. Fisher in *Sister Age* has a beautiful thought on this issue: "Children and old people and the parents in between should be able to live together, in order to learn how to die with grace, together." I suppose she's right. Dying surrounded by family wouldn't be the hard part for me. The hard part would be living with them and feeling I was in the way of their lives. Guess I'll need to wait until the time comes and decide then what's in the best interest of us all.

How do you feel about this?

_____

_____

_____

_____

Under what circumstances and guidelines would you be willing to live with your adult children?

_____

_____

_____

_____

Robotic Romeo

"The trick for younger family members is to help without feeling trapped and overwhelmed; the trick for older members is to accept help while preserving dignity and control."

—Mary Pipher, *Another Country*

I have an eccentric habit of stacking up magazines to read and letting them marinate for a year or two or ten until I get good and ready to read them. Then, like a hungry wood fire, I burn through them, slashing and hacking away at ads and peripherals (like those annoying subscription cards and perfume samples) until I have a stack of articles only. On a recent foray into my magazine stash, I came across a not-too-outdated article on robots in an issue of *Scientific American*. It seems some company "aims to raise capital to develop a version to serve as a companion and helper for the elderly." It's a robot called the HelpMate. It has arms, voice recognition, and stereo vision.

I began to imagine my elderly life with one of these things. It felt cold. There I am missing my grandkids or my husband and my HelpMate (I'll call him Yanni because I have a fantasy going about the young, long-haired musician in white silk) responds to my tear-inflected pleas. I tell his voice recognition chip that I'm lonely and he embraces me in his steely arms, gazing at me with the kind blue stereo-vision marbles he has for eyes. He feels cold. His little robot face presses against mine. My tears short circuit his whirring electronics. Brrrrrrr. Cold.

I worry that my kids and friends will think Yanni a substitute for visits with me. I imagine them taking Yanni off in a corner one Sunday afternoon and telling him how to behave after they leave. "Make sure she doesn't sleep past 10:00 A.M. and get her to take her red pills before lunch, and the green and white one with dinner." Oh God. Could this be my future? "And when she starts to reminisce about the old days, sit quietly without comment, nodding until she's done. Don't forget to look interested." Cold. "Oh, and when she complains about her children and how we never come to see her, tell her it was just yesterday they were here—she'll never know the difference, she loses track of the days anyway." A frosty future with a robotic HelpMate complete with empathic listening, steely arms, stereo vision, and programmed compassionate responses. Ugh.

I have a plan. If presented with this robotic sorry excuse for a companion, I will take my elderly self and Yanni on a shopping trip. I will dress him up in a dark, long-haired wig, white silk shirt, and tuxedo. Then I will take him for a tour of the Hawaiian Islands and spend every cent of my children's inheritance on hula lessons!

How do you feel about this?

_____

_____

_____

_____

_____

_____

_____

Unfinished Family Business

"Everyone has a stack of painful memories, rejections, disappointments, ridicule, sorrows over what might have been . . . we have a choice about whether we forgive others including our parents and heal ourselves or let the hurts go on festering."

—Betty Nickerson, *Old and Smart: Women and Aging*

One of the blocks to successfully moving into the second half of our lives is unfinished family business. A friend of mine, a more-than-middle-aged woman, has not spoken to her parents or siblings since she graduated high school. I don't know what caused the breach, but I have other friends who are very close to severing family ties because they get continuing aggravation instead of the understanding and support they want. However, leaving some of these issues unresolved can keep you stuck in the energy of the past forever; and going forward in your life, you're going to need all the energy you can muster.

It is probably best to stay away from ultimatums and demands that people are unlikely to meet. If family members can't give you the support you need in an area that is sensitive to you, try to find some aspect of your life you can comfortably share with them. In some cases where a bridge can't be built, you may have to create a new family. It's never too late to do so. Weathering the storms of life isn't easy, and loving relationships can be a lifeboat—a lifeboat you can build by choosing new "family members."

I enlisted a new family for myself when I realized mine wasn't capable of giving me what I needed. When I was developing my new family, I never directly asked anyone to fill the roles. I learned about each person's background and developed a plan to strengthen the relationship. I invited them into my life, sharing intimate details with each.

Although her circumstances were different from mine, consider what Roberta Russell says in her book *R. D. Laing and Me: Lessons in Love*, where she describes how she re-created a family after losing her family to divorces and death. "I carefully chose six people for my new family. One was a great teacher . . . another, an excellent father . . . and so on. I worked hard to give them what they needed—and to establish trust. Being reliable was key."

Acknowledging your anger and disappointment with family members is key to moving into a healing process with them. Many years ago my therapist helped me honor my anger, to make meaning of it all, and ultimately move toward forgiveness. Allowing room for anger allowed me to move to a place where forgiveness and understanding could be born.

What does it mean to forgive? *Webster's* defines it as "to give up resentment against or the desire to punish; stop being angry with; to give up all claim to punish or exact penalty." If we are to forgive, we must first surrender the right to get even. We then cease defining the one who hurt us in terms of the hurt that was caused. Keep in mind, there is nothing in this definition about the need to reach approval of the injurer's actions. If we forgive, we can also reach a point where we wish our injurers well—this act of forgiveness then becomes some kind of miracle after we've made meaning of the situation.

Being able to let go of negative feelings towards others is highly dependent on our ability to let go of negative feelings towards ourselves. When we have developed the ability to let go of our own past mistakes, to acknowledge our humanness, it is almost magical how effortless it becomes to let go of the mistakes of others.

No family connection of any kind would last if the silent reparative force of forgiveness were not working almost constantly to counteract the corrosive effects of resentment and bitterness. The wish to repair a wounded relationship, whether it takes the form of forgiveness, apology, or some other bridging gesture, is a basic human impulse. Forgiveness is not just a by-product of growth: The struggle to forgive can promote growth, and that is my point. We are meant to keep growing as long as we live.

How do you feel about this?

_____

_____

_____

_____

What unfinished family business is draining your energy? And what are you willing to do about it?

_____

_____

_____

_____

_____

_____

_____

_____

Creating a Family History

"As a older family member, you give your family a sense of heritage, tradition and continuity that only your generation can provide."

—Eudora Seyfer, *How to Be Happily Retired*

For many of us, there comes a point in our lives when we'd like to pass on at least a portion of our family history to the next generation. At my grandmother's 100th birthday party, my son, then ten years old, interviewed her on videotape, asking about her voyage from Sweden to the United States in 1913. He asked her to describe her life back then. This taped interview is of course a precious historic record of immense importance to my family. Although Grandma was somewhat confused about the details of her earlier life, and the videotaping process wore her out a bit, she seemed grateful for the opportunity to pass on this part of her history.

We naturally want some of our life story to live beyond us. At the same time, we are drawn to put our own lives into a historical perspective. The Internet offers a treasure trove of genealogical information like directories of surnames, adoption and birth records, cemetery and marriage records, military records, ships' passenger lists, census records, immigration records, and a lot more. You can even find family sites that offer family trees, wills, and photographs.

There's a helpful book, *How to Create a Video Biography* by Ira Heffler and Jerry Schneider, that contains advice on preserving family stories and images. The book addresses such things as being a good director and editor; there's advice for good sound and picture, and it includes sample interview scripts.

You can write out your story and pass it on. You can give your family and friends a portrait of how you see yourself and what you have brought to your family and the world. Try making an uncritical list of remembered experiences and life events. Write down as many details as you can about the memories. It may not be easy, but be honest—you need not share all details, but tell the truth about what you do choose to write. Writing this kind of honest memoir usually generates a sense of well-being and that can lead to new insights about one's life and an emotional resolution to some troublesome problems. As a helpful guide on how to go about this process, take a look at Denis Ledoux's book *Turning Memories into Memoirs*.

How do you feel about this?

_____

_____

_____

_____

Do you know where you fit in your family's history? What stories would you like to preserve for your descendants?

_____

_____

_____

_____

_____

_____

_____

_____

12

Our Friends

"This third act—from age fifty on—can be the best act. If people know that you see them . . . that you hear them, that you really are taking them in, then you will never be without friends."

—Nancy Friday, *The Power of Beauty*

I know that my good friends enrich my life. They make the good times better and the bad times bearable. They give me support and help keep me stay connected to what's important. They help energize me and reduce my stress.

Experts continue to tell us to increase our human contacts for a longer and less stressful life. They tell us that close relationships at home, on the job, and in your community can keep you calm and help boost your immune system. It's important to make regular connections with people you like, to stay in touch with old friends, and to attend meetings of community groups—to make connections part of our everyday lives. I try to schedule a monthly lunch with a friend and consider it an unbreakable appointment.

Even so, when I get overly busy with my work and my family, my tendency is to let my friendships with other women slide. I push them to the back burner and that's really a mistake, because women can be such a source of strength for each other. We intuitively find it easy to nurture one another. We need to create unpressured space where we can engage in the special kind of talk that women do when they're with other women.

As I approach my sixth decade, I want to make my friends more of a priority. And if I can be a support to others who may need it, that is all for the good. Perhaps that is what our community or, better still, our society needs. We can be a big support system for one another with enough arms for everyone who needs a hug.

The famed Nurses' Health Study from Harvard Medical School found that the more friends women had, the less likely they were to develop physical impairments as they aged, and the more likely they were to be leading a joyful life. In fact, the results were so significant, the researchers concluded that not having close friends or confidantes was as detrimental to your health as smoking or being overweight. When the researchers looked at how well the women functioned after the death of their spouse, they found that even in the face of this biggest stressor of all, those women who had a close friend and confidante were more likely to survive the experience without any new physical impairment or permanent loss of vitality.

The issues and concerns about aging point to the necessity of creating and maintaining support systems, the ability to make new friends as old ones die, the need to strengthen existing relationships, and to get involved in community affairs. The essays in this section will help you identify what type of friends are healthiest and how friendships change throughout life. The strength of our friendships and our connection to community become increasingly important as we age. Hopefully this section will help you prepare for a time when some friends will die and others will move away, and you'll need to make new ones.

This section encourages you to look at the value of friends and the support they offer as we age, keeping in touch with friends through the years, clearing out friendships that don't work (toxic relationships), and how friends can affect your health and longevity.

What Matters

"I like being with women who have discovered the joy of who they are, who know that what matters more than age is whether or not they are strengthening their creative spirits, living authentic lives."

—Gail Balden, in *Our Turn, Our Time: Women Truly Coming of Age* by Cynthia Black

The preciousness of life seems to matter more to me now, and good, intimate friends seem to matter more now than the superficial ones of my earlier years.

Ask yourself, "What matters?" What answers do you get? Does it matter that you have one more gray hair today, or that you have one more day on the planet to connect with those around you? Does it matter that you have the pain of arthritis in your elbows and arms, or that you have arms in which to hold a friend who needs a shoulder to cry on? Does it matter that you can't remember the things you used to, or that you remember how loved you've felt in your life?

What matters changes as we move into the second half of our lives. Giving back seems to matter more now. Shirley Mitchell in *Fabulous after 50: Finding Fulfillment for Tomorrow*, tells us that "after 50, we find the joy of giving back, of pouring into others, of returning and serving out of the rich storehouse of the knowledge and experience we have gained." I couldn't agree more.

You may be the most important person in someone's life today. Have you considered how even the smallest gesture of friendship can change the course of a life? Consider the enormity of this truth. Isn't what matters most, as you view your life from its second half, how much you've expanded your capacity for love? Friendship is one of life's most special gifts. Treat your friends with the respect they deserve. Friendship matters.

How do you feel about this?

_____

_____

_____

_____

In what way can you let a special friend know how much he or she matters to you?

_____

_____

_____

_____

The Company of Other Women

"The angels attending her that night felt little twinges of longing to be in human form, if for only a few minutes. They wanted to rock, they wanted to roll, they wanted to feel the peculiarly human feeling of having a perfect night in an imperfect world."

—Rebecca Wells, *Divine Secrets of the Ya-Ya Sisterhood*

On one of our "Ya-Ya" excursions to Plum Island, Massachusetts, I asked my good buddy, Patty Henderson, to comment on what it was like for her to be older in the company of women. Her enthusiasm was contagious. Here's her response:

"I'm in my fifties! After 40 years of what you're supposed to do—all the would-a-could-a-should-a—I finally got it! Women are miracles! Any woman who's made it to her fifties has a profound story to tell—by the mere fact that we are female. Just listen. It's a secret society. Every day you get another secret password. Pass it on and don't worry. This movement is bigger than you could ever imagine."

As a movement or one on one, our women friends are there at the births of our ideas and our children; they are there for the celebrations of our lives, the losses we endure, and the deaths we journey to and through. As Janet Quinn said in *I Am a Woman Finding My Voice*, "We are not passive observers of each other's lives; we help each other live them. Women friends. Womanfriend. I cannot imagine my life without them."

I don't know what would become of me if it weren't for the company of other women in my life. Women who are older offer me glimpses of what life can be in later years. Younger women offer an opportunity to share some of my hard-won wisdom and keep me in the swing of things. Last, and most importantly, the women who are in my age group, who are moving through the journey with me, are my comforters, my jovial companions, and my confidantes. One of my favorite authors, Joan Borysenko, wrote in *A Woman's Book of Life*, "I find myself learning from women in their twenties, and from friends in their seventies. Perhaps the most important gift of the feminine life cycle is the gift of one another."

Research shows that those who have strong social connections are healthier and live longer than those who lack them. In particular, having a special friend and confidante was especially beneficial. Other studies found that

Our Friends

socially involved people are less subject to depression and handle stress better, and get this—they're less susceptible to the common cold.

When I was up against some of the hardest times in my life, my friends knew I would survive, as I had so many times before. They listened to my truth and mirrored back for me who I was when I had forgotten. That's the joy of women's friendships. We hold one another up when we're down. We listen with our hearts. We are honest with each other and remind each other about our goodness and strength. We join in each other's grief and loss. And perhaps most importantly of all, we know how to have fun when we're together. BettyClare Moffatt wrote her wish for the future: "When I am an old woman, I shall laugh hysterically with other old women, as we help each other across the street."

I think too many of us keep potentially warm friendships from happening because we judge ourselves by Martha Stewart standards. Because we were brought up in another era, many of us feel that we can't have friends in to visit unless our house is spotless and we can provide a five-course meal. We need to relax and invite our friends to come for a potluck-style dinner and ignore the dust balls.

Sometimes the best thing a friend can do is to be loyal and understanding enough that you don't need to see them or call them or remind them you love them. Sometimes you just need friends to understand that you need to be alone. Growing old, really old, is part of life, and we must help each other do the best we can.

How do you feel about this?

_____

_____

_____

_____

Describe a particularly heartwarming experience you have had in the company of other women:

_____

_____

_____

_____

_____

_____

_____

_____

_____

_____

_____

Companions on the Journey

"My peers notice my bifocals, my old-age spots, my matronly abdomen, and soft pads on my hip bones, but they accept me for my understanding and companionship."

—Sarah Bierman, in *Our Turn, Our Time: Women Truly Coming of Age* by Cynthia Black

I think growing older with friends is fun. Their companionship can be especially valuable when they help you lighten up about the whole process. My friend Sari and I joke about having surgery to move the soft pads on our hip bones up to our shoulders to use as shoulder pads. My sister and best friend, Marilyn, and I joke all the time about how our old-age spots are one day going to connect to each other and give us the look of a year-round tan.

Good friends are such an asset, I can't imagine a life without them. I love what Patricia Lynn Reilly says in her wonderful book *Imagine a Woman in Love with Herself*: "Imagine a woman who values the women in her life. A woman who sits in circles of women who is reminded of the truth about herself when she forgets." We do forget from time to time who we really are and what it is we bring into this world. Friends who know us well and who are supportive by nature have no trouble reminding us of our value when we're down and out.

When we reach a certain age we are entitled to feel wiser, less constrained by what others think. We become less judgmental and more capable of

Our Friends 229

unconditional love—at the same time, we're tired of putting up with other's nonsense and unreasonable demands. We tell it like it is and have more of our authentic selves available to invest in friendships.

It's interesting to consider, but in the early to mid part of the 1900s, women weren't generally considered as interesting company as men. Barbara Sher in *It's Only Too Late if You Don't Start Now* implies that an interesting shift took place in the 1960s: ". . . we woke up, looked around and discovered a world full of fascinating women. Why didn't we see them before?" Well, I'm seeing them now, and appreciating them even more than I could have possibly imagined.

How do you feel about this?

_____

_____

_____

_____

List the names of your three most important companions, and why they are important in your journey of aging:

_____

_____

_____

_____

_____

_____

_____

Making New Friends and Cleaning Out the Old

"I think I can truthfully say that I have never had so many friends. They are not only interesting and stimulating, they are generous and uncritical. Most of them are women."

—Rebecca Latimer, *You're Not Old until You're Ninety*

Here's what is true: Not all friendships are good for you. Admit it, some friendships actually drain your energy and erode your self-esteem. Some have upset, disappointed, or betrayed you. It's not too late to let go of these unhelpful relationships.

A good friend is honest without being cruel. She is reliable, keeps her promises, and offers support when you need it. A real friend is not judgmental, is a good listener, and is someone you can have fun with. Toxic friends lack some or all of these characteristics. Why do we make such friendships? For one thing, no one comes into our lives bearing a label that says "promise breaker" or "fault finder." It can take time for a friendship to reveal itself as good or bad. We may hold on to a toxic friendship because we believe we won't at our age be able to make new ones.

Forming new friendships is key to healthy aging. Centenarians report that they have a remarkable network of nontoxic friends who care about them and offer help when needed. Not every contact has to be a close one. Even regular, friendly conversations with your grocery store clerk count. It might be helpful to rekindle old friendships from your childhood and young adult years. Having these people as part of your life in later years is sure to prove meaningful. Next time you're invited to a class, workplace, sport, or other reunion, make it a point to attend and make a new friend.

People with close, nontoxic friends live longer than those who lack them. Bet you didn't know that supportive friendships improve your chances with cancer. A recent study of ovarian cancer patients indicated that women with strong social support have lower levels of a factor that stimulates tumor growth. Solid, supportive relationships relieve stress, which lowers blood levels of stress hormones. Friends who truly care about you are more likely to cajole you into seeking medical help and take care of you. Think about the potential effects on your health of moving far away from longtime friends

Our Friends

after retirement. You'll definitely need to make new ones then. You may not realize until an emergency strikes that the good friend who would have come over at 4 A.M. isn't nearby.

You need to take a risk or two to make an acquaintance into a friend. Let them see you as you really are. Share something of yourself that you would not share with just anybody. Suggest spontaneous activities to do together. Listen to what matters to your friends. Ask for advice or help on a project. Tell them you like them. If you are annoyed, or think your friend may be, bring up the situation and work it out together.

Sometimes our own comfort can be found in giving comfort to others. A giving spirit increases longevity. A study done at the University of Michigan's Institute for Social Research found that "it isn't what we get from relationships that makes contact with others so beneficial. It is what we give." You boost the spirit of someone in a touchy situation, and you get to live longer.

How do you feel about this?

_____

_____

_____

_____

Think about your five closest friendships. Do these relationships uplift you or drain you? How can you surround yourself with people who bring you comfort?

_____

_____

_____

_____

_____

_____

_____

_____

When Friends Die

"When pain and fatigue wrestle, fatigue wins. The eye shuts. Then the pain rises again at dawn. At first you can stare at it, then it blinds you."

—Marge Piercy, from "When a Friend Dies" in *The Moon Is Always Female*

There's no easy way to deal with the inevitability of losing friends. If you live long enough, friends are going to die. You may even live long enough to have all your friends die before you do. Perhaps one of the best ways to deal with the loss is in a creative way. My sister dealt with the loss of one of her friends by writing this poem:

Liz

. . . Liz, I think of you . . . , especially
when trees are bare, December's empty arms
praising the sky . . .
I want to think of how things grow, not how they die
I want to remember the Magic Pan where you and I
would sit for hours, laughing, planning, scheming
about the usual stuff, hopes high
So, Liz,
I promise you, yeah, I really mean it, I've had enough . . .
when Spring comes again, and everything is fresh
I'm really gonna try
to lose the sadness.

—Marilyn Houston

You will never forget those friends who've gone before you, and with time, other friends will come to touch your life. Try not to close off the possibility for new, enriching relationships. And in the meantime remember, if you've lost a friend, you now have a personal guardian angel watching over you.

How do you feel about this?

_____

_____

_____

_____

Is there a creative way you can remember a friend who has passed?

_____

_____

_____

_____

Where Is Everybody?

*"I was looking at my address book. Just about
everybody in it is dead! I was thinking of putting
together a new address book, but I didn't like the idea
of leaving all those folks' names out."*

—Sarah L. Delany, *On My Own at 107*

When we were younger, death seemed distant and somehow impersonal. But gradually, or suddenly, as we age, more people around us die. In part this is because we know more people, but more than that, it's because we are older, as are our friends and relatives. Death becomes relevant, personal, close. Lives once unshakable are shaken by death, or by losses, the loss of dreams, the loss of friends, the loss of relationships, the loss of health or an ability to function.

In addition to the wonderful, same-age friends you've acquired, consider making some younger friends. This can be important to your welfare as you get older. We naturally lose old friends as they age. They don't all die. Some move away and retire in another state or another country, like my friend Maxine who moved to New Zealand.

Having younger friends will keep you more engaged with new ideas and more physically active and help you maintain a younger attitude and lifestyle for yourself.

Betty Friedan wrote that "most of my friends are younger . . . you need to make friends that are younger. I have to say that in the last couple of years, three of the men in my life have died, and the women are still going strong."

How do you feel about this?

_____

_____

_____

_____

Class Reunions

*"When I went to my fortieth reunion I couldn't help
but ask myself, who are those old people?"*

—Carol, 59

Does the idea of a class reunion bring up terror in your heart? I think women spend more energy on crash diets and fixing themselves up for these than any other major event in their lives besides their own wedding. What are we trying to prove? That we haven't aged a bit? Are we still trying to get back at the guy who ignored us all through high school? You know, the one you had a crush on so bad you thought you couldn't live another day without him? Or that skinny blond cheerleader who called you fat and ugly?

Despite swearing I would never ever do it, I went to the twenty-fifth reunion of my high school class. I hadn't seen most of those "kids" since I graduated. None of my old friends looked great, although of course I think I did. I dropped 20 pounds in preparation and made sure I wore my most expensive jewelry. Such pressure.

The same cliques were operating at the reunion. Those friends who were tight then were still huddling close together, eying and assessing the other attendees. I felt like I was under scrutiny.

I thought of some of the good times in high school. I remember the days when we wore strange clothes and listened to music that made our parents crazy. We trusted no one over 30 and shocked our parents by rejecting the accepted Establishment values. We were passionate and idealistic. By our sheer numbers, we defined our times. That was more than 30 years ago, and the baby boomer generation has officially reached middle age and then some. The idealism of youth has been exchanged for the need of a good 401K, an investment portfolio, and concerns over healthcare costs. Our drug of choice is now a potent over-the-counter pain medication. We never trust anyone under the age of 40, especially those young doctors. And hey, man, we are the Establishment.

How do you feel about this?

_____

_____

_____

_____

If you went to your high school reunion, what did it bring up for you?

_____

_____

_____

_____

The Yeah-Yeah Sisterhood

"Sometimes it only takes a word, a phrase, a drumbeat, a circle, a song, a room full of women in harmony together, to remind us of all that we are."

—BettyClare Moffatt, *Soulwork: Clearing the Mind, Opening the Heart, Replenishing the Spirit*

Once a year I join a small group of women on an adventure like no other I experienced in my younger years. Sari and Patty rent a house on Plum Island off the Massachusetts coast each year, and each year they create a space for us to join one another in a ritual of sisterhood. We design and make things that reflect our authentic nature. One year we made hats, using glue guns, bows, shells, and assorted other decorative items. When we posed for a photo wearing our hats I realized just what a bonding experience we had created.

Another year we made purses to wear with our hats. Again, out came the glue gun, feathers and beads and shells. One of our "sisters" bought outlandish muumuus for each of us at a thrift store and we posed once again as a group with our hats and purses as accessories.

The Next Fifty Years

Julie described her experience as follows: "I am the youngest of this group of extraordinary women. Precise age is not really an issue with us. As I look at each of these females, it's like looking into windows of what may or may not happen to me when I reach their stage in life. With all of them I see it as a privilege. I've been given a rare insight to my future. We all have very different careers, marital status, upbringing, size—and yet I feel such unity as a group. We all learn so many things from one another. Just being among them as a collective 'family' is the best learning experience for a fledgling like me. Because of them, I look forward to new journeys of age with whatever time I have left on the planet."

As Ruth Turk said in *The Second Flowering,* "It is easier to share joys and sorrows with those your own age who are going through the same kinds of experiences at the same time."

How do you feel about this?

_____

_____

_____

_____

Write down an idea for creating a bonding experience for a group of women that you know:

_____

_____

_____

_____

13

Our Play

"We are all little girls in aging bodies. No matter how old we are, we are still that little girl that skipped rope, roller-skated on the sidewalk, skinned knees, wore braids with barrettes or ribbons, and ate ice cream bars from the ice cream man."

—Jo Schlehofer, *Celebrate the Older You*

As we grow older do we need to grow more serious? Do we need to stop being playful and young-spirited? Ask yourself what gives you pleasure and delight? Have you forgotten? Did you leave your inner child behind at the playground?

Your need to play doesn't diminish with age. No self-help book, Indian guru, or bossy sister can tell you what will give you pleasure. To find what gives you joy, you have to divine it for yourself and listen for your inner child's urges. Each day I ask myself, "Have I done anything fun yet?"

We need to laugh at ourselves more and get out and play. Someone once wrote, "If you laugh . . . you last!" That's true. My 75-year-old grandmother knew how to play games like Parcheesi and canasta and how to get down on the floor with us and shoot marbles. My friends over 70, Len and Tita, once got together with a small bunch of friends to wander around silly in a supermarket like escapees from the loony bin.

I got an e-mail a few days ago that said, "You don't stop laughing because you grow old, you grow old because you stop laughing." That's very true. A sense of play and a sense of humor are essential to aging successfully.

This section urges the readers to put more fun in their lives, to develop a sense of humor, to seek adventure, to remain curious, and to take the needs of their inner child seriously.

Are We Having Fun Yet?

"When I was thirty, I had no clue. If I'd known how much fun, what freedom, would be found in these September years, I would've lied about my age and gotten here sooner."

—Lynne Zielinski, *Chocolate for a Woman's Spirit*

Did you know that the average number of times an adult laughs in a day is 15, and that kids laugh 150 times a day? When was the last time you had some good, old-fashioned fun?

I remember my grandmother skipping rope when she was in her sixties—just for fun. Remember skipping without a jump rope? Skipping burns almost as many calories as running and it's probably more fun. I even read somewhere that you can join a skipping club! On a recent vacation to Hilton Head Island with some girlfriends, we rented three-wheelers and rode around the island for a day like little kids. What fun we had.

If you aren't a naturally happy person, with very little effort you can cultivate pleasure. Creating pleasure is not beyond your control. If you take having fun and creating pleasure seriously, you will find ways to reorient your inner compass and change your thoughts and feelings. With a little effort you can shift your mood.

Rebecca Latimer wrote a great book called *You're Not Old until You're Ninety* in which she says, "Somewhere along the way I picked up the idea that if I refuse negative thoughts and emotions, if I smile rather than frown, laugh rather than cry, my mood changes entirely." I believe her.

I'm not talking about activities you could do in your sleep. And eating doesn't count unless you are truly immersed in the act of cooking, serving, and tasting. The pleasure in most rote activities, if there is any, wears off in about ten seconds. Rote activities don't get you to the state of sustained well-being I would call pleasure. Try cultivating activities that result in a state of sustained well-being. Experiment with activities that require attention, like learning a language, painting a mural, taking your grandchildren to the park. Lose yourself, forget about time, and come back feeling different. My friend told me the only time she could lose herself like that—say, by visiting an art gallery—was when she'd convinced herself it was work-related.

One 62-year-old woman I spoke to gets up at 6:15 A.M. to knit and listen to classical music before she starts a busy day of volunteer work. Another runs marathons on the weekends for the sheer exhilaration of it, and one 82-year-old takes piano lessons for the "high" of it. Have fun, just for the sake of having fun. Blow bubbles—the benefit is that you inhale oxygen, which is good for the brain. Play with pipe cleaners or Play-Doh (it's also good for exercising arthritic hands). Draw with crayons, paint with watercolors, and by all means, get a glue gun and make something.

How do you feel about this?

_____

_____

_____

_____

Name some things you've had fun doing in the past—could you do them now?

_____

_____

_____

_____

Can you think of some new ways to have fun?

_____

_____

_____

_____

Laughing Out Loud

"Zen practitioners, who savor derision as a way of life, believe that laughing out loud is the only way to reconcile our wish to attain enlightenment with our repeated failure to do so."

—Veronique Vienne, *The Art of Growing Up*

Could guffawing yourself silly actually be good for your health? It certainly can. In 1979, magazine editor Norman Cousins suggested that laughter was powerful medicine, and studies have proven him right. Frequent laughing, the harder the better, may lower blood pressure, increase protective antibodies, and even cut the risk of heart disease.

I read the following warning on the Internet: "It's bad to suppress laughter; it goes back down and spreads to your hips." Daily laughter is a health elixir. Fake it if you have to. There are about 100 laughter clubs in the United States where members perform exercises at health centers, nursing homes, schools, and corporations. To find a nearby laughter club, or to start one, visit www.worldlaughtertour.com.

An article entitled "He Who Laughs, Lasts" in *My Generation* (September/October 2001) quoted Dr. Lee Berk, a pioneer of laughter research at Loma Linda University School of Medicine in California: "We're taking laughing to the molecular level now. We're using the sophisticated tools of the twenty-first century to establish what the Bible told us centuries ago: 'A merry heart doeth good like a medicine.'"

How do you feel about this?

_____

_____

_____

_____

List some things that are guaranteed to make you laugh and do them:

_____

_____

_____

_____

A Sense of Humor

"I heard recently that the philosopher Alan Watts used to make himself laugh every morning for ten minutes as soon as he got up. I tried an abbreviated, three minute version of that exercise. The results? . . . I was in a better mood all day."

—Valerie Monroe, *O: The Oprah Magazine* (May 2001)

At 20, I remember my mother (then in her 50s) sitting next to me in my 1966 VW Beetle when the skies opened up. We were caught in a downpour. As I started the car, Mom said hurriedly, "Are your windshield workers wiping?" When I repeated back to her what she said, we both burst into uncontrollable laughter. Have you ever had trouble finding the word for a familiar object? The older I get, the more of a challenge it's become. I once told my husband I was putting the dishes in the garage—I meant to say "in the dishwasher." We got a good laugh out of that one.

The *Journal of Personality and Social Psychology* reported that women who had the biggest smiles in their college yearbook photos had happier lives, happier marriages, and fewer personal setbacks in the following 30 years. (Go ahead, check your yearbook.)

You may be tickled to know that it's okay to fake it. Put on a happy face, and your body, either hoping for the best or not knowing the difference, responds as if the expression were genuine. Smiling engages at least three major muscle groups, increasing blood flow to the face and thus helping to create a rosy glow. Who couldn't use that? Laugh wholeheartedly, the facial muscles get toned; get delirious and give yourself a serious aerobic workout and help your immune system at the same time.

Even the gentlest smile causes your eyes to moisten. The muscles around the tear glands are stimulated, causing your eyes to sparkle and shine. Draw back your lips, and your raised cheeks round out your face, softening it; the increased blood flow nourishes your skin. Try finding lotions at the makeup counter that promise those results. And the next time you have trouble finding a word or name, laugh at yourself and you may end up looking much younger.

How do you feel about this?

_____

_____

_____

_____

How can you put more laughter in your life?

_____

_____

_____

_____

Challenges and Possibilities

"At fifty, we are challenged by a sense of adventure, stimulated by the wit and irony of life. We see the possibilities of this 'second half' of adulthood that lies ahead, and don't back off."

—Colette Dowling, *Red Hot Mamas*

I wonder what Colette Dowling is presuming about the majority of us. I wonder how many of you are challenged by "a sense of adventure" and how many of you are gripped by fear of the unknown, stimulated only by the desire to stay young, stay beautiful, stay alive. As I write this, I wish you could tell me.

In your future and present do you see possibility or disability? Perhaps Dowling is trying to tell us that this is the way we *should* be and can be if we try. I don't believe we are *all* challenged by a sense of adventure. However, we can be open to the possibility. I don't believe we are all stimulated by the wit or the irony of life. Some of us are decked by it.

We all know what our challenges are. For some, aging is a challenge in itself. A challenge to stay vital, healthy, and interested in life. Perhaps even in the face of challenge we can be more proactive in seeking out the small adventures, life's sideshows. You know, the ones that aren't necessarily the main events. Make a habit of driving or walking down a different street each day, learn how to play the harmonica, or do like my friend Patty did—arrange for a tugboat ride. Add one small challenge, one adventure, into your life today.

How do you feel about this?

_____

_____

_____

_____

How can you put a bit more adventure into your life?

_____

_____

_____

_____

Wonder Years

"The return of 'wonder' in old age is illustrated in 'elder tales' down through the ages . . . showing older people apparently outrageous or foolish after years of being practical and predictable."

—Betty Friedan, *The Fountain of Age*

The way Betty Friedan describes "wonder" in the above quote makes it sound like a valuable pursuit for my later years. She also says that this "wonder" is "an essential element of wisdom." I agree.

Have you become predictable and boringly practical in your older years? Hmmmm? Is it time to plan some wonder-filled events? Valerie Bell tells us that "aging well takes some planning. It's so easy to lose focus, fail to stretch for the best life has to offer, and end life full of regrets."

Sit quietly for a period of time today and think back to when you felt a sense of wonder at a particular event or time or place in your life. Then imagine yourself doing that activity. I remember when a sunrise took my breath away. We were on vacation in Cape Cod and we drove the car to the beach at 5 A.M. We simply sat there listening to music in the car while that gorgeous fiery ball rose from its sleep. What a wonder.

I'm tired of being practical and predictable. Maybe I'll order a pizza at midnight on Tuesday. I'll run out to watch a sunset this week because I'm not going to wait for a vacation to do this wonder-filled activity. The Hudson River is five minutes from my home, where there is a beautiful park overlooking the river with hills that slope gently to the water. At 6 P.M. I will sit on my folding chair atop one of those gentle slopes, drink wine, read Earth poetry, and watch the Sun set the horizon on fire.

How do you feel about this?

_____

_____

_____

_____

Make a list of ways that you can exercise your sense of wonder:

_____

_____

_____

_____

Traveling Adventures

"Here I am, eighty-three years old, and I have just returned from yet another travel of discovery to the Greek Islands."

—Helen Hayes, *Helen Hayes*

You don't need to go all the way to Greece to expand your horizons . . . there is someplace interesting, even new, for you to explore within a day's drive of your home. A part of the travel industry caters to an older population's need for adventure. Even a simple trip opens us to our need for new adventure, in purpose and project, a new exercise for our bodies and our spirit in age.

If you don't want to join a tour for senior citizens, consider what these adventurous women did. Joei Carlton Hossack, 59, has been traveling on her own in an RV. Her husband died of a heart attack when she was 48 and she continued to travel on her own in their VW Westphalia. She's authored many books on travel. Her most recent is *A Million Miles from Home* in which she recounts her solo world travels. What an inspiration! My 60-year-old friend Ellen went alone to Club Med Sonora in Mexico to participate in the big tennis camp they have there. I have another 60-plus friend, Barbara, who took off on her own to see the United States in her ancient Volvo wagon.

If you're traveling alone and you don't want to go off on your own, see if you can find a travel service that specializes in singles. They can help compatible travel companions find each other. Safety guidelines for traveling solo:

- Leave a copy of your itinerary with a friend or relative back home so you can be tracked down.
- Read guidebooks and carry maps of the cities you plan to visit so you don't get completely lost.
- Check in with the U.S. consulate.
- Ask about trouble spots.
- Only stay in hotels or motels with interior hallways.
- Don't wear expensive jewelry or carry expensive luggage, particularly in a Third World country.
- Carry your money and passport in a money belt or pouch that you wear under your clothing.

Visit the World Senior Games, or play in them. More than 6,000 men and women athletes over age 50 participate each year in the games at St. George, Utah, around mid-October. Events include swimming, cycling, tennis, bridge, bowling, and horseshoes (to name a few). They also offer healthy lifestyle seminars and free health screenings (see www.seniorgames.net; or call 800-562-1268).

Is a disability keeping you home? Recreation vehicles with disabled access are now available from more than a dozen manufacturers with features like wheelchair lifts, wide entrances, roll-in showers, etc. But not all RV campgrounds have accommodations for the handicapped. Check out the Handicapped Travel Club at www.handicappedtravelclub.com.

Husband or partner keeping you at home? Consider what Carolyn Heilbrun said in *The Last Gift of Time: Life beyond Sixty,* "I have, furthermore, discovered that for those . . . long married, separate trips are a chance to be oneself, to acquire, through the temporary detachment travel can offer, a fresh view of marital life together."

If you were to have a traveling adventure, where would you go?

_____

_____

_____

_____

What steps can you take today to make it happen?

_____

_____

_____

_____

Juicy Curiosity

"If you have twenty years or more stretching out before you, now is the time to learn something new."

—Ruth Turk, *The Second Flowering*

In old age, curiosity can be an innocent exploration. Like children, we can be newly refreshed by our world. We can see things with awe and wonder, with new eyes. The task is to become curiouser and curiouser. To look at the world afresh before we leave it. Maybe you won't be successful in staving off some physical challenges like arthritis, but there's no need to let your mind grow rigid and inflexible.

Twelfth-century mystic Hildegard of Bingen counseled her devotees to be "juicy people." According to her teachings, to be "juicy" is to be a fearlessly joyous optimist, a troublemaker tirelessly afflicting the comfortable, a passionate lover of tasty food and good talk, "a frequent violator of the ordinance against indecent exposure of the heart, and a guerrilla in the insurrection against Dream Molesters everywhere." She wanted us all to be filled with wonder and curiosity, with lusty appetites and high spirits, to embrace life, liberty, and the pursuit of happiness.

Make an effort to stay interested in life. Jeanne Calment, who lived to be 120 years old, once said, "Always keep your smile. That's how I explain my long life. I think I will die laughing. . . . Everything interests me. I've had a fine life."

Stay curious, be juicy and inquisitive. Ask questions—when you go to a store that displays and sells pottery or art, ask how it was produced. Go to the library and research a topic you know little about. Buy an old telephone at a garage sale and take it apart—haven't you always wondered how they work?

How do you feel about this?

_____

_____

_____

_____

Name some things you're curious about and find the answers somewhere:

_____

_____

_____

_____

Our Inner Child Never Grows Old

"Because I was once a child, I am always a child . . . my past is part of what makes the present Madeleine and must not be denied or rejected or forgotten."

—Madeleine L'Engle, *A Circle of Quiet*

Do you wonder if you have an inner child? We are like trees. When you chop one down and examine its stump, you can count the rings of its life. Like Russian nested dolls, we have all of our younger selves there inside us.

Somewhere inside a mature woman is a little child who wants to create, to play, to be free, to let go of the world of doing, and just be. In *It's Better to Be over the Hill Than under It: Thoughts on Life over Sixty*, Eda LeShan wrote, "A nice little nap in the afternoon, with an arm around a teddy bear, followed by cookies and milk, feels just as good at eighty as it did at three." She also said, "Inside me there is surely a child I have worked hard to keep alive, to help me understand myself and other children."

After many years of being pulled in many different directions by spouse, children, biological and hormonal changes, and life, now my small child Self can reemerge, intact, after a long sleep. Long before I was a woman there was me, the child. With reference to aging, author Hilary Lohrman said, "This changing time is a recovery, not a diminishment of me."

You don't need to cash in one self for another. Children aren't allowed to rule the world after all. If we live long enough we will experience many, many selves. I'm trying to learn to accept all my selves, the new and old, the child and the adult, inside me, not as strangers but as friends.

Let's face it, it's a great release to let yourself go, to sing and dance, to play games, or whatever else takes your fancy, without worrying about what someone might think. Reactivating the creative, playful child that is still within is essential to successful aging.

Go to a park and watch a child play, and you will notice that children delight at such innocent simple things, and so can you. Tell yourself that you're never too old to do anything your body will allow.

I leave you with this thought written by Irene Claremont de Castillejo, author of *Knowing Woman*, "The old woman . . . needs to turn her natural receptivity towards the inner voices and inner whisperings, pondering on the new ideas which will come to her if she is attuned to her own inner self."

Write a letter to your inner child and give her permission to be part of your life:

_____

_____

_____

_____

_____

_____

_____

_____

_____

_____

_____

14

Our Work

"Your work is to discover your work and then with all your heart to give yourself to it."

—Buddha

Someone once said, "Work is simply the opposite of rusting away." I believe that's true, provided you work at something you were designed to do. When you engage in what you were put on this Earth to do, the activity is exhilarating and interesting. The work begets energy, health, and happiness and helps to deflect tension and stress.

I'll bet you didn't know that the concept of the "golden years" originated as a public-relations program designed to make 60-somethings feel good about their forced ousting from the workplace. In fact, retirement isn't a natural part of the human life cycle. It annoys me that "retirement" was, and still is, a social engineering experiment designed to move older, "useless" workers out of the workplace to make room for the young.

As a retiree or person nearing retirement, you now have the opportunity to go where your heart leads you. But you also can get lost or run in circles. To know where you're going and how to get there, you need a map. Even if you look forward to retirement, you're giving up an identity.

As a woman ages, a sense of urgency may grow as it becomes more important to do something meaningful and satisfying with the remainder of her life. Where do you go next? Art school? Computer class? Start a home business? The only reliable guide is your inner compass—a sense of who you truly are. In the grip of life's demands, making a living, serving a family's needs, it's easy to lose that sense of self. But it's always there—a thread of identity that runs from childhood through all the years following. Making good choices means discovering your true passions—who you are—what gives you true joy.

For many women past 50, work is still an issue, and for some it's an issue they never had to think about. This next section will help the reader explore what possibilities exist after retirement or in one's later years. You will also be asked to think about and respond to questions of doing what you love, volunteering as a choice, and whether or not you have a calling that needs to be heard.

As Lavinia Russ says in *A High Old Time,* "When death comes for me, I hope I'll be so busy working and laughing, I won't hear his knock. He'll have to break down the door to get in."

Reactivate Your Dream

"This is the real fear of becoming middle-aged: not death or decrepitude but the dread that you'll inevitably turn into someone else, someone who doesn't live an exciting life or have exciting dreams."

—Barbara Sher, *It's Only Too Late if You Don't Start Now*

Listen to your dreams and learn their language because your dreams are trying to remind you of what you've forgotten. Let them guide you. If your earliest career decisions were driven by the need to make money, or a life decision to be at home with your family, the second half of your life can be driven by the fondest desires that you set aside in your youth.

At some point, most women feel unfulfilled in their lives or their careers, no matter how successful they feel they've been. To revisit and reactivate your dreams without giving up what you have achieved so far, begin by imagining that you no longer need to win approval for being beautiful, strong, or successful. If the social and financial pressures of making money never existed, what would you have done differently?

Notice what you love—reading magazines, listening to music, playing tennis, being in the country. These "loves" are clues to your hidden desires. As a young girl, what did you dream of becoming? Many of your dreams may have come true already and some may not be important any more. The point is, you need to reconnect with your inner dreamer. Once you are aware of your dreams, you may be able to find practical ways to act on them.

Whatever dream you decide is worth pursuing, break it down into small, manageable steps and explore them one at a time. This gentle process will help you move closer to feeling satisfied with your life. It will also allow you to recognize early on that a dream may no longer be worth the effort it would take to make it so. A step-by-step approach will let you see that there are many different ways to enjoy your dream. For example, you can realize your dream to be a writer by taking classes in the evening . . . or by merely reading about what steps other authors have taken to get published. Taking a class would take less time to master while at the same time providing you with the fulfillment that comes when one takes a step toward their dream.

What dream would you like to reactivate?

_____

_____

_____

_____

_____

_____

What small step can you take today towards making it happen?

_____

_____

_____

_____

Doing What You Love

"Essentially what happens when you begin to do what you love is that you get a new employer: Spirit."

Sarah Ban Breathnach, *Simple Abundance*

I read in the *Los Angeles Times* that an 80-year-old woman broke her leg in a parachute jump. She started jumping when she was 75. This fearless woman is representative of thousands of venturesome women in America who have passed well beyond the half-century mark. They are blessed with good health and are determined to continue what they've always done, or what they've always wanted to do.

I don't enjoy the concept of mortality—or jumping out of planes, for that matter. However, thinking about the limited time we have on this planet focuses one's attention on how to meaningfully and effectively spend the days that are left. So here's the pivotal question: How does one discover one's own natural talents and apply them in today's world?

Amy, a 45-year-old mother and veterinarian, told me she thought about what she wanted to do all the time—sketch and paint—but was waiting until the kids were grown to do it. Other women told me they didn't have enough time to figure out what they would do if they had the time.

There are plenty of ways to lose your direction in life. For me it used to be shopping and chocolate chip cookies. But the "me" who takes over when I indulge isn't someone that I'm proud of. In fact, it's usually someone I'd like to strangle when I come back to Earth.

Human beings weren't created to live at a frenetic pace. The hectic tempo of the modern office may suit a caffeine-soaked brain, but it may also upset our internal rhythms. Often career selection is undertaken entirely from the mind's standpoint, and we end up doing things for hours every day (such as sitting in front of a computer screen) that further our cerebral ambitions but cause our backs to stiffen, our muscles to atrophy, our eyes to weaken. The body is not a machine external to us; its health affects our mental acuity and moods. When choosing a career path, we should give some thought to the question, what does our body want to do?

You've had rich life experiences, you've acquired an extensive array of interests and abilities. Based on your life experiences, ask yourself: Who are you? What do you like? What do you do well? By selecting job or career opportunities that fit your personal values, skills, and ideal work environment, you will achieve lasting satisfaction and a sense of self-worth through your work. What things interest you most? What skills give you the most satisfaction and energy?

Start where you are and begin your future now. Create a sense of safety, increasing creativity, uncovering purpose, and staying motivated. Take stock of your present options and create a vision for your future. When you feel discouraged, talk to a supportive, interested friend, keep a journal, honor your body, and reward yourself daily.

Consider creating a bridge between your spirituality and your life's work. This means taking the essence of who you are and what you believe into your work space. If kindness, patience, honesty, and generosity are spiritual qualities that you believe in, make every effort to practice them in what you do.

Now ask yourself, what did you want to be when you were a little girl, before someone insensitive told you it wasn't possible and that no one makes money doing it?

_____

_____

_____

_____

Do You Have a Calling?

"We can live for years unaware of our hearthungers and their growing insistence until by mid-life we become famished. And then if we still have not awakened to the truth of how far we have run from who we were created to be, we 'sell out' and find ourselves groveling."

—Sarah Smith, *Mid-Life: Coming Home*

Do you have a "calling"? It doesn't necessarily mean a career. A calling is about your vocation, whether it is work, relationship, lifestyle, or service. It's about the search for personal meaning, which is a major developmental task of aging. Your heart may be calling you to do something (become self-employed, go back to school, volunteer, leave or start a relationship, move to the country, change careers). Your soul may be calling you to be something (more creative, less judgmental, more loving, less fearful).

You may feel that insurmountable obstacles are getting in your way. Many women hesitate to answer an authentic calling in midlife because they're caught between the financial reality of raising children and/or caring for aging parents, between the circumstances of their lives and creative choice. If you have it in your heart to play the piano, start a business, paint a picture, write a poem, or sing a song, then find a way to do it; don't let anything stop you.

Remember that you were born with the potential for the unfolding of your true self. If you deviate from that truth, you interfere with the intention of something far greater than you are and as a result, you run the risk of developing discomfort in your body and psyche. In fact, the symptoms of anxiety might be regarded as a message from a powerful force within you that wants you to be yourself.

Most women yearn to know their purpose in life. Perhaps your calling has to do with service to others. We come into life with nothing, and we leave it with nothing. Truth is, we can't take what we acquire and achieve with us. The most important thing you can do with your life is give to others. To be of service means you will ultimately feel purposeful. Whenever you feel lost or unsure, remind yourself: "My purpose is about giving. I'll direct my thoughts away from me and spend the next few hours looking for ways to be of service to someone or something else." We feel purposeful when we serve someone or something beyond ourselves.

Maybe your answer to "what is my calling?" will come gradually, as it did for English psychologist Joanna Field, born at the turn of the twentieth century, who said in *A Life of One's Own*, "I began to have an idea of my life, not as the slow shaping of achievement to fit my preconceived purpose, but as a gradual discovery and growth of purpose which I did not know."

As a final comment on this issue, I leave you with some wisdom from one of my favorite authors, Helen Nearing, who at 89 wrote *Wise Words for the Good Life*: "The universe is immense and gorgeous and magnificent. I salute it. Every speck, every little fly on the window salutes the Universe. Every leaf has its meaning. I think the Universe is expanding—it is experiencing and accomplishing. And we have the opportunity to add to its glow."

How do you feel about this?

_____

_____

_____

_____

If money and time were no obstacle, what would you be doing with your
life?

_____

_____

_____

_____

_____

_____

_____

_____

_____

_____

_____

The Entrepreneurial Spirit

"Age teaches us it's our duty to be and do what we love."

—Marsha Sinetar, *Don't Call Me Old—I'm Just Awakening!*

Think you're too old to risk becoming an entrepreneur? Why shouldn't you open your own business? At your age you have a lifetime of practical experience. If you have good energy and a financial cushion to tide you over until your business catches on, you could do just fine. And, you've always wanted to be your own boss. Do you have what it takes to succeed as an entrepreneur?

There are five principles that make for successful entrepreneurship: experience at an early age (working for other entrepreneurs, starting a small business as a child, etc.), finding niche opportunities, building a strong team of associates, making friends with bankers and suppliers, and understanding financial statements. And one other attribute that women especially have an abundance of—intuition. Women entrepreneurs also tend to be more interested in self-fulfillment than in money and power, which adds to their success rate.

As with so many things in life, your attitude will determine whether or not you'll be a success as an entrepreneur. You have to be able to stay motivated through ups and downs in whichever business venture you embark upon. You have to trust in your decisions and think positively. Your attitude will also rub off on those around you.

Regardless of your age, you may or may not be able to do all the work yourself. You must be able to put a certain amount of confidence in those you'll be working with. And you won't be able to delegate to others if you don't believe they are capable of handling their jobs. You need the ability to take on a certain amount of risk. Keep in mind that many things won't get done unless you do them yourself. When you're on your own, the buck stops with you.

Should you own your own business? Keep in mind that more than 50 percent of small businesses fail within the first year. Before you take the plunge, ask yourself these questions to ensure that you are suited to the task:

• Do you need supervision to work?

• Running a company means living with financial risk. Business ownership typically means working for long-term growth, not next week's paycheck, so do you need security and stability?

• Are you willing to work nights and weekends?

• Many businesses entail long hours, which can put a strain on your personal life, so is your spouse supportive? His life will change if you have your own business, so make sure you talk it over. Be sure to talk with your family about your feelings toward your business and how you feel about them so they don't feel overlooked.

The worst that can happen is that your business fails. So what? At the least you will have learned a lot. Perhaps what you learned in this venture can be applied to a new business opportunity. Be realistic. You can't expect to receive a regular paycheck for a while. Can you stay sane when you don't have a guaranteed flow of income? Money may be very tight in your start-up years. If you're looking merely to supplement your retirement income, you might want to consider taking a part-time job rather than setting up your own business. If you decide to start a business, be sure you've put away enough money to live on during the slow times.

Find the right business for you, one that fits your lifestyle and personality, one that is a good match with your talents and experience. Being your own boss can put a strain on your health. Make sure you find ways to alleviate stress, like regular exercise, taking time off for family and friends or just letting loose once in a while by doing something wild and enjoyable.

Find out if you'll need help. It's important to decide whether to work utterly alone or start your venture with others. Don't overlook the value of writing a detailed business plan. You need the plan as your guide and you will also need the plan if you want to raise start-up funds. Check your local library for helpful resources.

How do you feel about this?

_____

_____

_____

_____

Have you ever had an idea for a business? Write that idea below:

_____

_____

_____

_____

What steps would you need to take to make this business a reality?

_____

_____

_____

_____

Working Retirement

"I think the term 'retirement' . . . is much too negative . . . 'recreatement' sounds much more encouraging for that last and best third of one's life, which can be filled with newness."

—Helen Hayes, *Helen Hayes*

Today, as people stay healthier and are more active, many choose to work past the retirement age fixed by society's expectations or social security. Some of us simply enjoy working because it creates a sense of fulfillment. On the whole, we're a generation of women who are better educated and more health conscious than our parents were, and we're altering the concept of aging and retirement. A lot of us are still working, and in fact many women age 65 and over are planning to keep on working as long as they can. We may need to work longer than we had planned to survive economically. One good reason to stay in the workforce is that retirement savings, pensions, and Social Security payments may not be enough to provide the comfortable lifestyle we want.

While longevity makes it possible for more older workers to stay on the job, it also makes it more necessary. The number of very old workers is growing, mostly because of the stunning growth in the number of older people. When the United States was born, just one of every 40 people was over 65. Today, one in seven is.

We can work for money if we want or need to, or we can give back to society in some way. The most youthful and interesting people I know in retirement are those who are not concentrating primarily on themselves. If and when you do retire from a paid job, a new world of volunteer activities opens up. Nonprofits frequently need and welcome older volunteers because they appreciate their skills and know that they're reliable.

Longevity will most likely bring you choices about work. It's important to think about those choices and what you'd most like to do in your later life.

How do you feel about this?

_____

_____

_____

_____

What kind of work do you envision for your "retirement" years?

_____

_____

_____

_____

Too Young to Retire

"The idea that one should retire never crosses my mind. I hope I'll always be writing and physically active."

—Elinor Gadon, writer and scholar

We used to associate midlife with retirement and achieving that great golden dream of traveling around the country and reading all the books you didn't have time to read. Many of us have now arrived at midlife and all I can say is, thank God it isn't like that. There is so much more to do. In her inspiring book *On My Own at 107*, Sarah Delany wrote, "I don't see why folks should retire at sixty-five. I retired at seventy myself and looking back on it, I bet I could have kept teaching for a long, long while yet."

As the baby boomers reach retirement age, the growth of the workforce will slow sharply or stop, while demand for workers will continue to grow. By the year 2011, available jobs may outnumber workers by more than 4 million—rising to 35 million by 2031. Thus there will be more opportunities in the future for older women to have second careers if they want them

At this age I'm looking to older friends for inspiration. Do I want to retire like Len and Tita, high up in the mountains in their Swiss chalet-type log home near one of their married sons, surrounded with grandchildren? He's working as a part-time minister in two local churches, and she's reading to herself, reading to the grandchildren, doing crafts, and running a bible study once a week. Lots of homemade cookies for visitors, lots of running on Sundays.

Or do I want to retire like Maxine and Jim, six months in very affordable New Zealand, and six months in very expensive, tax-burdened Westchester County, New York, near some of their family and friends? He will open and manage a theater and will continue his meditation practice; she may continue some kind of work in the investment, financial planning field or open a muffin shop. They both love to travel and will make time for it.

Or do I want to retire like John and Sheila in the beautiful house on the coast of Maine that they rent out part of the year? When they're not in Maine, they live in their mortgage-all-paid-for house in New Rochelle, New York. She's a full-time professor and writer; he's a part-time, retired clergyman invested in social action projects. Back and forth they travel from house to house with a walk or two around Europe thrown in, along with lots of packing and unpacking and lots of driving.

So what is retirement anyway? Mary Baker Eddy was still the head of the Christian Science Church at age 89, and Coco Chanel was still CEO of her fashion company at the age of 85.

How do you feel about this?

_____

_____

_____

_____

_____

_____

_____

_____

_____

_____

Too Old to Get a Job?

"The idea that we are used up at sixty-five . . . is patently ridiculous. Why waste the experience of a lifetime?"

—Joan Borysenko, Ph.D., *A Woman's Book of Life*

You think you're too old to walk into a business and apply for a job? You're not. Millions of women over age 50 are taking up new careers, especially in areas that welcome mature workers. Work has no upper age limit. In fact, about 255,000 women in their seventies or older are still on the job.

Some work because they have to, but many work just to keep themselves feeling involved in life.

With the expectation of greater longevity, a lot of our future generations will be less likely to follow the traditional linear life plan—12 or more years of education, followed by working full time for 30 years or so, and then retiring. What if we could intersperse work, education, and leisure throughout our lives?

Older women who find a job that gives them cash and contentment are the women who know what they like and what they enjoy. They've found more than cash and contentment. They've found freedom.

By law, if you want to work, you can't be denied a job, a promotion, or any job-related benefits solely because of your age. Of course, this doesn't automatically guarantee you a job. As a practical matter, older workers may find younger workers are hired more readily than they are. Contact the Equal Employment Opportunity Commission (EEOC) (800-669-4000 or www.eeoc.com) if you have questions or concerns.

To get started, it's probably a good idea to call one of the temp agencies that trains and places older people in full- or part-time positions, such as Manpower, Kelly Services, or Olsten's.

Here's another idea. If you're retired and haven't worked in some time and are interested in doing some kind of job or starting a new career, take a look at the Occupational Outlook Handbook at your local library. The Handbook is updated and published every two years by the U.S. Department of Labor and contains descriptions of about 250 jobs—earning potential, training and educational needs, skills required, working conditions, and other facts.

When you fill out a job application, don't give your date of birth. Employers can't ask your age and you don't have to tell. Never write that you've been fired. Stress your accomplishments first. Skills are more important than pedigree these days. Remember that skills can come from outside the workplace. If you stopped working to raise a family, list relative activities such as your ability to multitask, budget, and organize. Volunteering can also provide notable accomplishments. The one page limit is a myth. It's hard to get 20 or 30 years of accomplishments on one page. Remember, 50 to 70 percent of people still get their jobs by networking. You can also get help on the Internet: see www.monster.com or www.hotjobs.com for good resume tutorials.

How do you feel about this?

_____

_____

_____

_____

If you were to apply for a job, what kind would it be? What skills do you bring to the table?

_____

_____

_____

_____

What Now?

"About three years ago, I found myself in that old familiar depression. I was turning 50 and mourning the loss of my youth. Who was I if I was not young?"

—Sally Fields

At every age, you have the opportunity to star in your own adventure, and you can decide if it is an adventure or a chore. Every age offers something you haven't experienced before (and I'm not talking about wrinkles and arthritis).

Sometimes our life's purpose and success sneak up on us unexpectedly, as with Liz Smith, columnist and TV journalist, who said, "The best thing that happened to me in old age was that I got to be successful after I was about to retire."

You have choices. Do you want to stay involved and engaged and look for ways to continue contributing to the world? Or do you want to follow conventional wisdom and fall back on the model of dependency? Do you find yourself spending a lot of energy lamenting your youth that you could be putting into your next venture?

How do you feel about this?

15

Our Finances

"As a group, we're markedly different from previous older generations who pinched pennies and saved them all."

—Joan Rattner Heilman, *Unbelievably Good Deals and Great Adventures That You Absolutely Can't Get unless You're Over 50, 2005-2006*

Those of us over 50 control most of the nation's wealth, including half of the discretionary income (the money that's left over after essentials have been taken care of). At this time of life, often the children are grown and mostly on their own, the mortgage has been just about paid off, the house is fully furnished, and the freedom years have arrived at last—or so the experts say.

Betty Friedan in *The Fountain of Age* found in her interviews with women that at the same time they were "opening to new adventure in age," there came the loss of some economic security—or, as she says, social status through widowhood or divorce. Okay, she's right. Few of us will escape the challenge of financial woes. But what else is new? As women, haven't we been the ones with the clever ideas around budgeting and stretching a dollar until it snaps like a rubber band?

Let's face it. Life is chock full of uncertainties. You don't know how long you'll live. You don't know what investment returns you'll earn. You don't know what inflation will be down the road. You don't know if next year will be a bear market or a bull market. Few of us want to deal with the subject of finances—myself included. But anyone who's been down and out at some time in their lives (including this author) will tell you that the lean time was also a time of great resourcefulness.

To be honest, I wanted to leave this section out of the book. I just didn't want to deal with the topic. Financial issues are not easy to face no matter what age you are and no matter what your circumstances might be. It is never too late to take stock of what financial assets we have and to become more aware of how we are currently managing our financial resources. We need to plan for change and find the information that will assist us in carrying out our plans.

This chapter will only take a broad look at those legal/financial general topics we must consider as we age, and it is by no means inclusive. I hope to help you lighten the emotional load by guiding you to take an honest look at your relationship to money and happiness, social status and security; how you can create enjoyable ways to live on less. I've also included some provocative questions and ideas on how you can help your children and your parents financially.

Getting Advice

"Growing older means learning to become good at giving up in some areas to gain new strengths in others."

—Katie Funk Wiebe, *Border Crossing: A Spiritual Journey*

Oh, I just don't want to write on this topic today. I have a gnawing feeling in my gut that just won't quit. About three months ago I made an appointment with a financial planner—a woman I trust. My husband and I promised to assemble and give her our vital financial information so she could work up an analysis and give us some recommendations. Every time I think I'll sit down and get it all together, the anxiety builds and I run to the refrigerator to visit my food friends. Cheesecake never asks you about your financial future.

To top it off, I just finished reading an article by Terence Reed, author of *The 8 Biggest Mistakes People Make with Their Finances before and after Retirement*, in which he says:

Mistake: Not putting your plans in writing.
Mistake: Being unrealistic about your exposure to risk.
Mistake: Neglecting to do "dignity planning."
Mistake: Closing the door on long-term-care insurance.
Mistake: Failing to understand the goal of estate planning.
Mistake: Stepping into tax traps that trip up retirement planning.
Mistake: Assuming you're too old for life insurance.

Too many mistakes to live with, and the article didn't even include the eighth one. Now I'm going to spend my sleepless nights wondering about that.

Okay, I need help. We all do on these matters. I'm promising myself I will call the financial planner next week and tell her about my anxiety. Maybe I can get her to come and hold my hand a bit more. I can't be the only woman she's ever met with financial anxiety. I'm sure it has something to do with denial. I just want to feel peaceful about it all and that sounds like a worthy goal—peace.

How do you feel about this?

_____

_____

_____

_____

If you haven't already, what small step can you take this week to getting the financial advice you need?

_____

_____

_____

_____

Giving to Your Kids While You're Still Alive

"Women have to understand. . . . It's not your duty to pay for your child's education. It is your duty to give your child an education about money."

—Suze Orman, author and personal-finance editor, CNBC

Here's another sore topic. I love my grown kids and I'd give them the world if I could, but it seems as if every time I turn around, they need a loan for something important. I don't remember asking my parents for more than a couple of hundred dollars to put down on my first car, a 1967 Volkswagen

Beetle that took me a lot of years to pay off (new it cost $1,979). After their help with the small down payment for my Beetle, I don't remember ever going back to them for more. Has the world changed so much? Doesn't it seem that our adult children are more financially dependent than we were?

When you loan money to your adult children, assume you will never be paid back. Even well-meaning children will put you at the bottom of their list of creditors. Check with your financial advisor because the government can change the rules on you; however, as of this writing, you can give a gift of $10,000 to anyone tax free every year—$20,000 from a couple giving jointly. If you have the means, consider family loans as gifts. This prevents hurt feelings and strained relationships when the loan is not repaid. And while from an income tax standpoint, writing off a bad loan is preferable to making a gift, it may invite IRS scrutiny, so put it in writing.

As for leaving money to your children when you die, here is one caution. If, for one reason or another, you disinherit a child, you guarantee that the child's only memories of you are bad ones. If you need to acknowledge in your will that the relationship between the two of you was not the best, then leave your child something, even if it is not as much as you left other children. The risk is that if one child is left more than another, despite the fact there may be good reasons for this move, you may ruin their future relationships with one another.

When it comes to money and your adult children, I say consider giving what you can while you're alive and when it's appropriate. If you can afford to, why not give them some happiness and security while you're alive to see it?

How do you feel about this?

_____

_____

_____

_____

_____

_____

_____

_____

Helping Your Aging Parents

"The great lesson to be learned in this last developmental stage is acceptance. That lesson well learned brings serenity. In the end, everything is about love."

—Mary Pipher, *Another Country*

About 7 million of us care for our aging parents. I'm not one of them. Both of my parents have passed on, so I won't have to face some of the difficult issues around finances that many of you will.

You might have to do some of the financial work for your parent, e.g., pay bills or balance the checkbook. To help maintain their dignity, allow them to sign the checks or review what you've done. If you live far away and can't monitor the bills easily, ask the utility and telephone companies to put emergency third-party notifications on the accounts. If any bills ever go into default, you would be notified before service is shut off. Many companies will do this for elderly account holders.

If you suspect your parents are being financially exploited, don't adopt a wait-and-see approach. Try to be vigilant about signs of exploitation like large withdrawals, unauthorized ATM use, or a new name added to the account. Ask your parents to let you run a credit check on them every so often to see if any new accounts or lines of credit have been opened in their name without their knowledge. Visit regularly if you can. If you live far away, have a friend drop by or hire a service. Ask your parents if they will allow a financial adviser to conduct annual checkups of their portfolio and insurance policies to prevent trouble.

You may be reluctant to bring up the issue of estate planning with your parents because you don't want to appear greedy. However, you might ask them to go with you to an attorney with the idea that you want to update your own will. Remind them that if they haven't made provisions, the state will apply its own formula for distribution of the estate and the state won't respect your parents' wishes.

How do you feel about this?

_____

_____

If your parents are still living, in what ways would it be appropriate for you to help out financially or otherwise?

_____

_____

_____

_____

Living Well on Less

"Many of us live below the poverty line but manage finances with a genius that would earn distinction in the board rooms of the nation."

—Betty Nickerson, *Old and Smart: Women and Aging*

Are you one of those people who hates to be called a "senior"? Get over it. You may be getting older, but once you hit the designated birthday—sometimes only your fiftieth—you become eligible for an astonishing number of great deals simply for having lasted so long. Whether you are offered these discounts out of respect for your age or because someone realized it was a major marketing tool, you'd be crazy not to take advantage of what's available.

I know a few women who refuse to ask for a senior citizen's ticket at the movies or any senior discount whatsoever, and I think that's foolish. We're all getting older, and as author Frances Weaver says, "You're just ahead of the pack, right now." Carry proof of age with you. Join AARP and they'll send you an ID card. Get a senior ID through your local Office of the Aging. This card entitles you to a wide array of discounts. Don't be afraid to ask for discounts wherever you shop.

Here's my advice: Don't wait for anybody to volunteer information about your special privileges. Be bold. Ask if there's a senior discount. Some hotel chains offer half off the regular price—just about every lodging chain and most individual establishments in the country will give you a break if you're over 50.

Being frugal is not the same as being cheap. In *Your Money or Your Life*, author Vicki Robin says, "Trace the word 'frugality' back to its Latin roots and you may be surprised to learn that it does not mean being cheap. It means enjoying the virtue of getting good value from everything you have in life."

Here are some ideas of my own and others that I've gathered from a variety of sources:

- Don't go shopping unless you really need something. Buy only what you can afford.
- Take care of what you have and don't throw out anything if it is still usable.
- Do it yourself. Stop trying to impress people.
- Get by with one car and keep it as long as possible. Shop around for auto insurance and drop unnecessary coverage.
- Rent out space in your home.
- Learn to shop the Goodwill, Salvation Army, garage sales, and thrift stores in your area.
- Try not to spend coins smaller than a quarter for routine purchases. Put the coins in a jar. With this "found money" you can get a massage, invest it, or take a class.
- Find a low-interest credit card.
- Join a co-op to buy food in bulk. Buy meat when it's on sale and freeze it.
- Choose basic clothing styles that can be dressed up or down and build your wardrobe around a few colors that compliment you.
- Clip coupons: find them on the Internet; shop at stores that offer double coupons.
- Revive the lost art of letter writing or, better still, send e-mail instead of making expensive long-distance calls.
- Call the local utility company for an energy audit and take advantage of its cost-saving advice.
- Consider low-cost entertainment options such as early-bird dinners, college theater presentations, and inexpensive adult education classes.
- Make gifts more meaningful by passing on an item you already own such as jewelry or a knickknack.
- Take books, audiotapes, videotapes, and music CDs out of the library rather than buying them.

Here's one of my personal favorites. Before I buy anything, I imagine it sitting on a garage sale table. You'd be surprised how many times I've put an item back on the shelf after considering what I would be selling it for in ten years.

How do you feel about these suggestions and ideas?

_____

_____

_____

_____

Which suggestions do you find yourself resisting?

_____

_____

_____

_____

Add your own ideas below:

_____

_____

_____

_____

Money and Stuff

"Another bonus to growing older is the increased ability to appreciate what one has, and a decreased interest in spending all that time and money shopping."

—Mary McConnell, *Still Dancing: Life Choices and Challenges for Women*

I can't say it enough times: understand what's going on with your money. Unless you've been diagnosed with mental health issues or some other disability, don't give the job of primary money manager to someone else in your family. If you're 60 and suddenly find yourself alone, you'll feel anxious and overwhelmed if it's been 25 years since you've had anything to do with your finances. If you're married, find out now what your husband is doing, and how he does it. Know each other's passwords and PINs. If there's a safe-deposit box, for heaven's sake, know where it is and where the key is.

When in doubt, seek the advice of a trusted professional who is willing to hear your concerns and field your questions, no matter how silly they might be. How do you find a trusted professional? Ask some friends for a referral and check credentials with a related financial organization.

When you meet with a financial advisor, some of the questions you will want to ask are: When my husband dies, what financial/legal steps should I take? What happens to my assets when I die? Do I need a living will? Should my will be updated and how often? Will I have enough to live on? How can I start a savings program?

You'll want to have your important financial documents in a place where someone can find them if you become ill or die—documents such as your will, bank account information, a durable power of attorney, a medical power of attorney, insurance policies, and investment documents.

If you feel a bit daunted and overwhelmed by the subject of finances, you're not alone. Midlife and older women, especially those who have engaged in limited paid work or whose marital status has changed, are likely to have had little financial experience or education. Don't despair. You really don't need an advanced degree to achieve financial literacy. You simply need the courage to ask questions and find a professional to guide you.

How do you feel about this?

_____

_____

_____

_____

Planning Retirement

"Rehearse your retirement. Decide what sort of retirement life you want, discuss it with your spouse and try it out about five years before you plan to stop working."

—Christina Povenmire, CFP, Financial Planning Association

Staring us right in the face is the fact that we have a "longevity bonus" of roughly 30 years or so past retirement. The challenge as we move into the next century is, what are we going to do with those bonus years? How are we going to spend them, and with what resources?

We all know that retirement can be stressful. If you are now suddenly spending more time with your husband, you may have disputes about how to spend your time and your money. It's helpful to begin planning retirement years before you retire. Agree in advance how you will adjust to retirement, from spending all your time together in activities like travel, to splitting chores, to both getting part-time jobs. Review finances to project how much you will have to spend, and agree on what to spend it on. Retirement will come much more easily if both of you have already agreed on how to handle both your time and your money.

The goal-setting stage of planning is a time to dream and visualize your future. Do you want to travel? Move to a different place? Spend more time with your grandchildren? Launch your own business or a new career? Take up a new sport or hobby?

If you expect to play golf every day, take a two-week vacation at a golf resort and do just that, to see if you would enjoy doing it for years. Since you and your spouse will probably be spending more time together in retirement, take a week off together and spend it at home, without any specific plans.

Calculate how much money you will have to live on during retirement, and try living on that amount for a time. You may find full-time retirement impractical, and part-time work may be necessary. The postretirement letdown can come from financial as well as emotional causes, a realization that your finances aren't providing the retirement you had anticipated. Be honest in your retirement planning, so you know exactly how far your nest egg will carry you.

The honeymoon phase of retirement ends six months to two years after you've taken the initial steps. And if you haven't prepared for what happens next, you may become depressed, feeling unimportant or unappreciated because you aren't doing anything meaningful or significant. It's very important to prepare for the end of the retirement honeymoon. Start by making clear, long-range plans to go back to school, develop a second career, or involve yourself in community service.

It is often the husband who makes the retirement plans, and the wife, who often outlives her spouse, must struggle to make them work. Remember that if you've worked most of your life, you will have the same problems in retirement as your husband. Many homemakers find the transition to be more difficult than someone who has worked outside the home. Women who have been homemakers all their lives must insist on being a full partner when the working spouse retires.

If you are married, the retirement phase of your life involves both of you, and any planning has to be done jointly. You need to agree on when to retire, where to live, the financial resources that will be needed in retirement, and how each will deal with the emotional letdown that comes with the end of the retirement honeymoon.

Anticipate the phases of retirement and plan ahead for each. For most people, retirement will consist of four phases, with different comfort zones required for each.

First, as I mentioned, there is the transition or the honeymoon phase, when you're first getting used to the idea of being retired. The task of this phase is to build a structure that will sustain you when the honeymoon ends and the "posthoneymoon" letdown begins.

Then comes the active-living phase, when you're healthy, vigorous, and over the posthoneymoon letdown. Now you might be able to do the extensive traveling you always hoped to do or go back to school.

Next is the slowing-down phase, when you're still pretty healthy, only now it's harder to get around. You might use this time for catching up on such long-deferred activities as organizing your family photographs, writing your memoirs, telling your grandchildren how you lived as a child. You might still want to travel, but tours will be more your speed.

Fourth, there is the assisted-living phase. Let's face it, none of us wants to think that we will someday be dependent on others for help. Most of us will need some assistance when we become old and truly infirm, but don't spend your retirement years obsessing about it.

You will probably want to spend some considerable time considering these issues, but to get started, use the space below to write the answers to these questions: What do you want to have, to do, to be, and to see during your retirement years? How will you continue to feel worthwhile and valuable to society? Will you continue working part time or volunteer for a charity? What will your finances be like in retirement?

_____

_____

_____

_____

_____

_____

_____

Wealth and Happiness

"There are so many other ways to feel rich in your later years that have nothing at all to do with financial wealth."

—Debbie, 74

I'm happy when I wake up to blue skies in the spring. There's no admittance charge for that view of the sky. I'm happy when I smell homemade bread baking (costs less than store bought). I'm happy when I see the smiles on my grandchildren's faces (priceless). Of course, I'm also happy when I can pay my bills.

Then there are the days when I sit down to pay my bills and run scenarios in my head that bring me way down, like, what will I be able to afford when I'm 75? Will I have to give up my occasional trip to Chico's for a new T-shirt? Will I be eating Cheerios and peanut butter for three meals a day?

A Harvard University study found that if you want to stay happy, healthy, and active into your 80s and beyond, "your attitude toward yourself and others matters more than your cholesterol level." As I see it, wealth is a poor predictor of happiness and health. The women that I spoke to who were happiest in their later years were not necessarily wealthy. In fact, as our culture has become more affluent, we haven't gotten any happier. Research says that even though Americans earn twice as much in today's dollars as they did in 1957, the proportion of those who say they are "very happy" has declined from 35 to 29 percent. What does that tell you? We spend so much of our first 50 years trying to achieve and accumulate wealth and material goods, and it doesn't buy us any long-lived happiness.

As we age, we can find another way to calculate our worth other than that of money earned. At 56, I'm so much more aware of what really matters. The designer handbag that I thought was so important to have when I was 30 sits on a shelf in my closet collecting dust as a reminder of how many hours I had to work to buy it. What was I thinking? Most likely I was hoping that someone would notice my wonderful bag and think that I had "made it."

I imagine that, like so many American women, I won't be able to afford everything I'd like in the future, but what in the world is it that I need anyway?

How do you feel about this?

_____

_____

_____

_____

Part IV

16

Looking Forward

"Paradoxical as it may seem, to believe in youth is to look backward; to look forward we must believe in age."

—Dorothy L. Sayers

Best-selling author Gail Sheehy once said, "I'm aware of looking for my future self and I think that's something women in their fifties begin to do." It is certainly something my sister, Marilyn, has done as she describes her experience of meeting with and accepting her future self in her poem:

The Message

I wanted to take the old woman's hand in mine
touch future-perfect version of my unmet self
to comfort her . . . and me
restore life-force through her bony hand
to reach her heart . . . and mine
as if through sheer belief my love
could touch, restore faith, release the lock
of time upon her heart . . . and mine
She passed and turned to look at me
driftwood in her eyes
a knowing smile released her face
as if she could read my intention
as if we had broken the code to acceptance
as if she understood my wish
for her . . . and me
From a stranger on a crowded autumn train . . .
an unexpected gift
waiting to be opened.

As we move into the future, we will be redefining aging. After we battle the cultural attitudes that try to define us and attempt to stall us out, we will be staying involved in life in any way we can—volunteering, working, growing, creating, discovering, and enjoying our lives.

What will our world be like in the next ten to 50 years? If we don't get run over by a bus, we have a good chance of seeing old age. Diseases, accidents, and illness will be treated in very advanced ways. In the years to come, replacing diseased or worn-out body parts will be as routine as replacing auto parts today. Scientists predict that a scan of your genetic structure will detect symptoms or susceptibility to particular diseases. Nanobots, minuscule robots, will deliver medications to affected cells to prevent or treat disease. Or they will clear clogged arteries or repair damaged tissue. You'll be able to have your vital signs tested by machines at the drugstore and send the results to your doctor via the Internet for analysis. Implanted biochips will monitor your vital signs, alerting you or your doctor to an impending crisis.

As we work to balance our physical, emotional, and spiritual lives, navigating the years ahead will require us to keep an open mind about technological advances. Imagine you are seated in a special chair that senses if you're cold or uncomfortable and adapts accordingly. Then you pull a bubble screen down around you. As you sit relaxed and comfortable, your computer/entertainment center will be programmed to teach you any language you want, produce a jazz bass line to go with your computerized melody or let you play a round of virtual reality golf.

Even as we look forward, we must not leave the richness of our past to atrophy on a dusty shelf. We can learn so much from revisiting where we have been. In *It's Only Too Late if You Don't Start Now*, Barbara Sher reminds us that we shouldn't forget about the past and live only in the moment. "That would be like forgetting the books in your library, when every read makes them come alive again." It is easier to get through midlife and move forward if you take the time to stop, look back, and take an inventory of all those times you didn't listen to yourself. At the same time, you're not meant to regret and dwell on the past, but rather to grow from it.

We know that our life expectancy has increased to the point where large numbers of us will have 30, 40, or even 50 more years of life. Many older women experience seemingly contradictory things such as increased emotional strength, physical energy, and an eagerness that is coupled with feeling constrained from within and from without. In this guidebook we have faced transitions in our relationships with ourselves, our families, and our communities. We've realized that there is no set chronological point at which old age begins, and that creativity is not just the domain of the young. In these pages,

The Next Fifty Years

we've explored our health and our wholeness on more than one level, addressing our feelings as well as our intellect, our bodies as well as our minds.

On the issue of aging, the next years will be an interesting time for our society. When a growing percentage of the population lives past 100, we will see what happens to the psychological and spiritual direction of our culture. The first step toward successful aging begins with a realistic assessment of our current life situation and the challenges that will undoubtedly confront us in the future. The choice not to choose is the choice to live irresponsibly. If we do not choose our activities and attitudes with clear judgment coming from a courageous and realistic assessment of our lives and circumstances, we fall into choosing unconsciously and poorly, and will pay a hard price.

In the pages that follow you will be asked to consider the future in a variety of ways, including any dreams you still have for yourself, what it takes to start over after loss or disappointment, and what you need to let go of in order to move forward. You will be asked to consider and respond to what it means to accept your humanity, what changes you can make to enhance your life, what you've learned from your past, and ways you can inspire the younger generation by leaving a lasting legacy.

Future Dreams

"Joy comes out of simplicity. Simplifying your wants, needs, desires. It comes out of balance and order. But not out of giving up . . . your dream."

—BettyClare Moffatt, *Soulwork*

I've decided that old age will be a new experience for me. I've never been there before, and I want my old age to be different from my youth, not just a continuation of it. Just because I'm older doesn't mean I have to stop dreaming about the future. Perhaps the dreams you have at night when you are sleeping will give you some clues to what you'd like to do with the rest of your life. Or perhaps daydreaming will show you the way toward an expression of your authentic self. Marsha Norman, author of *The Fortune Teller*, wrote, "Dreams are . . . illustrations from the book your soul is writing about you." Think about your dreams. What is your soul writing about you?

Anne Sexton once said, "In a dream you are never eighty." I like that. Keep on dreaming, dreaming about your future, and the future of the world.

As you live longer, you will start to see the earlier dramas, treasures, and goals of your life as part of a learning curve, a learning experience that's been neither wonderful nor awful. In looking back over my life, I understand that actions I once thought praiseworthy actually caused harm, and things I judged harshly simply indicated an innocent narrow-mindedness at the time. As I grow older and perhaps wiser, the meaning of life rests more on my willingness to see that outside goals were not as important as I thought them to be.

It is the endless pursuit of career goals, personal wealth, fancy vacations, and public recognition that focused our energies on things that didn't turn out to matter as much as we thought. Gay Gaer Luce, founder of the Nine Gates Mystery School in Petaluma, California, said it this way, "When we are freed from the quest for success by outside measures, the quality of our day-to-day lives again becomes important to us. And this growing attitude will bring a marked—and delightful—difference to American life in the future."

Writing something down makes it real. Your words about your future goals and dreams become magical messengers as your hands inscribe the thought in your brain as well as on paper. When you use this method to seek your goals, something special happens—it works. Through writing, the subconscious lets us know what we want.

Write a paragraph that describes your dream for the future:

_____

_____

_____

_____

_____

_____

_____

The Next Fifty Years

The Freedom to Change

"As some people age, they grow nostalgic for yesteryear. Not me. For me, this really is the best of times. Not too bad to be sixty-six and feeling at the top of your form, is it? I am just hitting my stride. Oh, and it gets better and better."

—Della Reese, *Bonkers Magazine* (October/November/December 1998)

It is said that to everything there is a season. You've been one way your entire life until now. Whether we like our lives as they are or wish for change, the first universal law is that nothing stays the same. This nonnegotiable fact propels us through a lifetime of difficult leave-takings and exhilarating renewals. The most significant changes are wrought by the awesome force of time. Without any concerted effort on our part, time will make us wiser and gentler.

Sooner or later we find that we lose our breath walking up a hill that once posed no challenge. We glance at the reflection of an aging woman in a store window and discover with shock that we are that woman. Although time will impose its natural changes on your body and soul, you still have control and freedoms at this age that you never had before.

We all have two lives: the one we learn with and the one we live with after that. If the one life you have been living with is begging for change, now is not the time to be cautious in exploring new parts of yourself.

Is it too late to change? Write down in as much detail as you can how you would like to change and evolve during the next years of your life:

_____

_____

_____

_____

_____

_____

_____

_____

_____

_____

_____

Feeling New Again

"I have enjoyed greatly the second blooming that comes when you finish the life of the emotions and of personal relations; and suddenly find—at the age of 50 say—that a whole new life has opened before you."

—Agatha Christie

In *On My Own at 107*, Sarah Delany reports that "one day in early spring, just when it seemed winter might never end, I ventured outdoors and was greeted by a wondrous sight: Bessie's crocus plants were peeking through the snow." Sarah's sister Bessie, over 100 years old at the time, had planted the crocuses many years before her death. Now their flowering reminded Sarah of a philosophy they had shared. Bessie and Sarah, sisters who were devoted to each other and their professional careers, never gave up on themselves or each other. They managed to feel that each new day was a blessing, a chance to be "new" again. In the sisters' first inspirational book, *Having Our Say*, they describe how they keep fit doing yoga each morning. Yoga at age 100-plus! There are days when just moving my mouth to say the word "yoga" is all the exercise or mental stimulation I get.

Now, if you're going to embrace the concept of feeling new each day, perhaps the symbolism of a crocus "peeking through the snow" will inspire you as it did me. Think about it, crocuses start out as wrinkled little turd-like orbs, sleep frozen in the earth for months of cold weather, yet have the audacity to live through it and timidly peek through the ground to display their fragile flowers once again. Think about that.

So you may be feeling a bit like a turd. Go for a walk and notice something beautiful along the way. Get your hair done and ask the hairdresser to massage your neck. Get yourself a touring bike and go for a ride. Pick apples at an orchard. Notice the trees budding in spring, help out at a children's home. Try a yoga class for mature women. Look for ways to feel new again.

How do you feel about this?

_____

_____

_____

What can you do to change your outlook on life and feel "new again"?

_____

_____

_____

Doors and Windows

"Doorways are sacred to women for we are the doorways of life and we must choose what comes in and what goes out."

—Marge Piercy, *The Moon Is Always Female*

Every life event is a door to discovering more about yourself. No matter what our age, we need to look for these doors because they are there, waiting for us to find them. This is the beginning of the rest of your life and a good time to ask how many doors are still left for you to open, which window views have been obscured and need cleaning. Windows and doors have opened and shut, gotten stuck, and at times the key to unlocking them is lost altogether. As you move into the second half of your life, which ones will you shut, which ones are stuck? Which doors will you open, which ones need a new key?

Try to remain hopeful like Joan Rivers, who said in *Don't Count the Candles*, "I have become my own version of an optimist. If I can't make it through one door, I'll go through another door—or I'll make a door. Something terrific will come no matter how dark the present."

We have heard that the eyes are the "windows of the soul" and "when one door closes another opens." Joseph Campbell told us that when you follow your bliss, doors you never knew were there will open to you. You are more than your crow's-feet and you are more than the wrinkles on your eyelids. Doors will continue to swing open when you keep a positive outlook, when you follow your bliss.

Today, begin to make plans for the rest of your life, one window, one door at a time. Make an effort to discover which doors are still open to you, which ones will need to be locked shut, what kind of windows you want to look through, and which offer you a better view toward the second half of your life.

How do you feel about this?

_____

_____

_____

_____

Make a note of which "doors" you'd like to close and which "windows" need a cleaning:

_____

_____

_____

_____

Becoming Human

"What separates the self-lovers from the self-haters among us? Are their bright sides brighter? Are their dark sides darker? Not necessarily. People who love themselves have an innate sense of their own humanness."

—Marie Lindquist, *Holding Back*

I'm human, all right! I know because some days are easier than others. I know because I don't sleep as well as I used to, or the "senior moments" get the better of me and I can't find the humor (human) in it. Some days every bone crunches and scrapes against the others and going upstairs seems a feat (or a defeat). There are days when the grouch that lives inside my throat says one too many "ughs."

Of course, there are days when I'm bright. When the brain is crisp and functional, when the creaking bones aren't quite as noisy. When I love that my eyes are working well enough (with glasses of course!) to read the good books and to see the bad movies. That my eyes may have trouble with the phone book, but can still read the poems. That my eyes can hardly distinguish "1 cup" from "1 tbs." in the cookbook, but see well enough to stab the chicken with a fork, cut it with a knife. I love that my bones can be warmed by sipping English breakfast tea, that my teeth can still munch through a whole bag of trail mix. I love that I am able to write what I'm seeing or feeling some days, and that I can hear music and laughter.

Today I will not dwell on the times I have so little patience with myself that I want to evaporate into the heat of the sun. I love me, I love me not, I love me, I love me not. I'll turn up my light a little brighter. I'm human and that's all right with me.

How do you feel about this?

_____

_____

_____

_____

Are you having trouble accepting your humanness? Why?

_____

_____

_____

_____

Harvesting the Past

"I am like one sent away to gather the harvest, and now returning, baskets full. Enough, I think, to sustain me in the autumn and winter that is still ahead. Until I am gathered, at the end, into the Creator's own great harvest."

—Hilary Lohrman

The word "harvest" brings to mind images of a horn of plenty—of fruits and vegetables spilling out, overflowing with bright, autumn colors holding the promise of abundance and nourishment. I believe harvesting our past for what sustained us holds the same promise.

I remember conversations with a 72-year-old friend of mine who was writing her memoirs. She remarked that as her short-term memory seemed to be misfiring, her long-term memory was firing up. Much to her amazement, she was recalling events she had not thought of since they occurred. She wrote about her firsts—her first love, pet, home, experience of death, disability, triumph—and found her life rich with resources she could use going forward.

When you harvest your past, you will undoubtedly come across an expanded frame of reference that offers your life a cohesive spiritual meaning. In *A Woman's Book of Life*, Joan Borysenko tells us that "the need for an older woman to tell and retell the stories of her life is no idle preoccupation with the past." She says that this is a vital process that helps us come to terms with events and experiences.

My twenties and early thirties were a challenging and intense time. At that time I was a divorced single mom living on a very limited income. I see now that I gained a resourcefulness that may be needed in the future when

I'm faced with living on retirement income. Although tough, those lean days 30 years ago were filled with joy and appreciation for the small things. Dinner out was an event planned and looked forward to for weeks. There was the anticipation of finally bringing home the sweater put on layaway for three months, and the Christmas my daughter and I cut out from catalogs those items we couldn't afford to buy but wished we could give each other. We pasted them into wrapped gift boxes we put under the tree. As a result, I'm not afraid of living on a budget as I age—a different kind of abundance awaits me.

In *Journey to the Heart*, Melody Beattie says, "Value what you've learned in your past. Each lesson has led to the next. Every person and event in each part of your life has been invaluable in shaping and forming you—in creating the person you are today."

Harvest your past with an intention to enrich your life today. If you choose to see only what you haven't accomplished, the material things you never had, the roads you think you should have taken and didn't, then you are not harvesting the past for what nurtures you. Instead you are pulling in negativity and filling your silos with moldy grain. Today, reap the rewards of your story, choose to gather in your personal wealth, celebrate the harvest.

Make a list of people, places, events, and experiences that helped shape who you are. Use the space below to get started (you'll probably be able to fill a whole notebook):

_____

_____

_____

_____

_____

_____

_____

"Harvest" a story from your past and tell how it is enriching your life today:

_____

_____

_____

_____

_____

_____

_____

Get on with Living

"I'm reading more and dusting less. I'm sitting in the yard and admiring the view without fussing about the weeds in the garden."

—Written by an 83-year-old woman to her friend

Let's get on with living, with becoming intimate with our lives and what makes us happy. We may be overlooking the best things in life because we're focusing too hard on what doesn't matter. Many of us aren't truly living. We put off doing what would make us happy. Notice how often you say "someday" and "one of these days."

For example, how about all those things you've been saving for a special occasion? How long are you going to save your good china for some special event? Isn't today a special event? Why deny yourself the luxury of eating a meal on a dinner plate rimmed in 24 carat gold?

What about your "dress-up clothes"? When was the last time you wore your velvet slacks just to go to the movies? How about that blue silk blouse that's been hanging in the back of the closet? Wouldn't it be fun to wear that to the supermarket? On a trip to the library, can you see yourself pulling out your library card from the hand-beaded clutch you use once every five years when you attend a wedding?

What are you waiting for? How about the $75 bottle of perfume sitting on the dresser top waiting to be used for a special night out? Why not spray some on before your next trip to the hardware store? Take off your beat-up sneakers and wear your best shoes to meet your friend at the diner for pancakes.

I've made a promise to myself that I'm not going to waste another day. I'm reading those books I bought two summers ago and decided I'd read someday. I'm going shopping in my closet for dress-up clothes and I'm going to wear them. The special occasion I've been waiting for is happening now at the picnic table in my own backyard. Tonight I use the lace tablecloth. Tonight I eat a hot dog on the good dishes.

How do you feel about this?

_____

_____

_____

_____

Name three things you've been putting off doing or using:

_____

_____

_____

_____

How can you get on with living instead of waiting for life to happen?

_____

_____

_____

_____

Starting Over

*"Tell me how you reconcile desire with the reality of
an aging body. . . . Tell me how you start over
again and again, rise like a phoenix from the ashes,
resurrect yourself, and go forward."*

—BettyClare Moffatt, *An Authentic Woman: Soulwork for the Wisdom Years*

I remember thinking that the car accident I had just before I turned 50 was the end of life as I had known it. Unable to get my injured brain to function at it always had, I had to let go into a new way of being. I was forced to start over. I decided this close call with death was an opportunity to start over in a dramatic way. Perhaps I was being forced to let go of the younger, frantic, overworked, ten-balls-in-the-air self and start a new life pace. Mary McConnell, author of *Still Dancing,* said it best when she wrote, "The women who seem most vital in their later years often are women who have been divorced, widowed, or have suffered some similar crisis in late middle age that got them moving in new ways."

Car accident or not, at 50-plus we begin an entirely different part of our lives, and for many of us it's a part so different we hardly recognize it as being connected to the younger ones. It's so new. Life is new and we find ourselves starting over again.

Oprah Winfrey said in O: *The Oprah Magazine,* "As I see it, if you have ignored anything in your life you should have paid attention to in this life—this second, moving into the third act—is the time to do it. This is the time to start living your life."

Today, no matter what went before, women at 50 can decide what their next 30 or 50 years will be like. Instead of seeing 50 as the start of the end as our mothers did, we can choose to see it as a new beginning.

BettyClare Moffatt wrote that "the alternative to aging is leaving the planet. But as we do age, as we do move from green shoot to ancient nurturer, we choose again and again. Daily we choose."

How do you feel about this?

_____

_____

_____

_____

_____

_____

_____

A Support for the Young

". . . this hour of union with the old woman soothed her like music, like chords lightly touched in the evening. . . . She leaned against the old woman's knee as a support, a prop, drowned, enfolded, in warmth, dimness, and soft harmonious sounds."

—V. Sackville West, *All Passion Spent*

One of the greatest legacies we can leave is to have been a source of comfort for someone. As with Sackville West's character, the idea of soothing someone "like music," of being the place someone can come to lean against for a while, that my "old woman's knee" could be a support for a wounded soul—that who I am could provide a soft place to fall for a younger person.

The young are faced with so much today. They woke up one day in September 2001 to a world that had changed. A world that wasn't making much sense anymore.

In *A Woman's Worth*, Marianne Williamson tells us, "In our fifties we should be able to shine. People in their fifties are like full-bodied wine. In our sixties and seventies, we could, in addition to shining, start teaching others, those coming up after us, how to do what we have done." Give it some thought. Is there an organization in your town that could use a volunteer to mentor someone younger? Is there someone in your family, or your friends' families, who would benefit by your spending a little extra time listening to them? What about your own children and grandchildren? Are you a support and a soft place for them to be vulnerable and not judged?

I know that when my day includes a moment or two of helping or inspiring someone younger, I feel purposeful and more alive—as if some of their "youngness" has rubbed off on me. We have a duty as the wiser ones to offer our "knees" as support for our younger ones who can benefit from our "music."

How do you feel about this?

_____

_____

_____

_____

In what way can you be supportive to someone younger?

_____

_____

_____

_____

Living Forever

"I know I don't want to live forever—but I wonder what it would feel like."

—Anne, 51

A range of new findings is snapping into focus the prospect of a radically new science of aging—one that points toward the possibility of lengthening human life span by the relatively simple manipulation of a small number of genes. Excitement is mounting among biologists that the secrets of longer life will be discovered in the next two to three decades. Many biologists say it's conceivable that human beings could be rejiggered to live 150 to 160 years. Suppose you had a choice: Would you live out your expected life span—currently 80 years for a woman—or live 122 years, the longest documented human life?

For all the excitement, science doesn't yet have answers to the most fundamental questions about aging. For example, what are the biological factors that determine why we age differently? Nonetheless, scientists imagine that aging will be slowed either by surgery such as stem cell or gene therapy, or by taking a pill. We may one day be able to replace tissues and organs in our bodies with new ones made from our own cells. Of course, controversy rages. Some anti-aging efforts are being outlawed and all are being hotly debated. Should society license drugs against aging? At what age should people take them? At 18, 45, 65? What side effect to the body and/or the brain should be considered acceptable?

To answer these questions, researchers say we are probably 20 years from having a grasp of all the biology we need to enable us to make a rational decision about clinical trials on people.

Roy Walford, a pathologist and author of *Beyond the 120-Year Diet*, believes that humans might one day achieve immortality by changing how we eat. The diet he proposes will make people skinnier, more tired, unable to sit on hard chairs, less interested in sex, and hungrier. Yeah, I want to live like that forever.

Perhaps in the future it will be mandatory to have some of your cells banked (maybe at birth) and when you get sick or start having aches and pains you'll say to your doctor, "Doc, I need some cartilage because my hip joints are worn and painful. Could you order up some new cartilage for me?" Then a few months later you get an injection into your hip and instantly get a new lease on life. I suppose there's no reason we can't go on replacing our parts indefinitely.

We could become the first generation to control our own destiny, a position human beings have never before occupied. Some say if we can prevent old age, why not? If we can prevent suffering, why not? Why not live to see your grandchildren and their children grow up?

If you could live a very long life, would you? Why?

_____

_____

_____

_____

_____

_____

_____

_____

Leaving a Legacy

"If I do have a fantasy, it's in the role of young people coming to me and my being able to share with them some of the wisdom I've gained."

—Jane Goodall, in *On Women Turning 60* by Cathleen Rountree

We older women have a particular hard-won wisdom that we've gleaned through consciously processing the experiences of our lives. What are we going to do with this wisdom? Play canasta on Tuesdays, bingo on Wednesdays? Get our nails done? We have an opportunity, and a responsibility on some level, to be mentors for the younger generation. It doesn't always go smoothly, however. Someone once said that mentoring is like dancing where the partners move with grace and sometimes step on each other's toes.

First of all, mentors do not impose doctrines and values on the people they mentor in an attempt to clone themselves. Instead, they foster others' individuality, applauding them as they struggle to clarify their own values and discover their authentic life paths. We bless them in the heroic, worthwhile, and difficult task of becoming more than they would have become alone. We encourage them by saying, "So what if you made a mistake—you can start again," or "I did the same thing when I was young." In the pursuit of leaving a lasting legacy, cultivate the art of attentive listening, carefully portioning out comments and thoughtful questions. Real communication occurs when you've taken the time to tune into the other.

In this exchange, communication is a two-way process from which both parties benefit. You will find the younger person's vitality will rejuvenate and invigorate you as you share in their energy and fresh ideas. Meanwhile, the younger person receives perspective and a readiness to bridge the past and future.

Go slowly; trust takes time. If you insist on dispensing wisdom regardless of someone's readiness or willingness to receive, the younger person won't be receptive. Don't impose your own knowledge, but try to evoke their own innate knowing. Resist trying to impress them by claiming to be perfect. Be your searching, tentative, very human self instead. Respect and call forth their uniqueness. Don't attempt to create an ideal follower based on your own hopes and ambitions. Recognize that mentoring has its seasons. Be willing to let them graduate from the work that brought you together.

The legacy you leave can also be as simple as passing on your story or your treasures. Martha McPhee described her grandmother in "Blue Bowl of History" in *Utne Reader*. She recalled that "her house was her art, a monument to her life. Each treasure revealed a portion of her biography. She was determined that I know her stories, as if by learning them I'd carry her legacy forward, assuring her a certain immortality."

The happiest older women are those who readily give of themselves to younger generations. We all have unique gifts to share and pass on. Before you can capitalize on your uniqueness, you must have a good idea of what it is that makes you different. So, ask yourself—in what ways am I unique?

Take an inventory of your gifts and skills and list them here:

_____

_____

_____

_____

_____

_____

_____

What knowledge would you grieve for if you died without passing it on?

_____

_____

_____

_____

Where will you look to find someone to mentor?

_____

_____

_____

_____

For Future Generations

Consider the possibilities—robots to clean your arteries and your rooms. Implanted computer chips that hold your medical records and lockets that contain your bank records. Surgery performed in your living room in front of a wide-screen televised operating room and luxury suites at hotels on other planets.

Women in the new century won't be disappointed with the upcoming array of show-stopping, smart technologies intended to improve our everyday lives, but we may not be able to figure out how to use them! While we yearn for the convenience and aid of high-tech marvels, I don't think many of us would be willing to give up our hardback and paperback books for words scrolling down a screen or a live concert at Carnegie Hall for the virtual-reality version.

Consider this: technology may extend human life spans by years, even decades. However, do you really want to be married to your spouse for 80 or 90 years? Artificial intelligence experts say that computers will be able to calculate and "think" as well as the human brain by 2020, but do you want to own a machine that's smarter than you are?

Scientists predict that there will be something called an "intelligent room" that will have walls that can "see" and "hear" you, then "speak" to you in response to your requests. Oh no. No hiding out in secret with your box of Oreos without an intelligent room scolding you. Here's one I like—they tell us that most household equipment, from TVs to toasters, will respond to voice commands. Guess you'll have to watch what you say to your microwave! They also say that smart cupboards and refrigerators will automatically reorder food that runs out. Can you imagine never running out of ice cream sandwiches—heavens. Electronic wall paper will let us change the color and pattern of your walls instantly (isn't that something some of us accomplished in the 1960s with drugs?).

Besides technological advancements, what do we want to leave to future generations of women? With or without scientific advances, through our actions, we will create a new image of age for generations to come. We will show them that age can be free and joyous, that it's possible to live with pain and loss, that it's important to say what we really think and feel. We will show them that we know who we are, that we know more than we ever knew we would, that we're not afraid of what people think of us as we move with wonder into an unknown future. In this moment in time we are helping to shape the future of aging for every generation of women that follows after us.

The developmental task of the second half of life has to do in part with generativity. Generativity is an adult's concern for and commitment to the well-being of future generations. In other words, creativity that lasts. We have opportunities to be generative in many different ways—as parents and grandparents, teachers or their assistants, mentors, leaders, friends, neighbors, and volunteers. Giving birth to a child is perhaps the most fundamental form of generativity. But people can "give birth" to many different things—from starting a business, to writing a poem, to painting a work of art, to coming up with a new solution to an old problem. Generativity is also about caring for the next generation. The task is to accept that we won't live forever, and to seek to leave behind a positive legacy for the future.

Generativity is a process and a journey and is always mutually beneficial. Travelers on this road develop the virtue of caring, which paves the way to a rewarding second half of life. This valuable quality focuses on concern for others beyond the immediate family. It demonstrates practical concern for the younger generations and the quality of both social and environmental conditions that we are passing on to them. Caring can also be expressed through the development of thoughtful products, careful systems, quality literature, insightful art, concern for the planet's well-being, and more. The choice to practice healthy caring in the second half of life expands our essential nature and bestows gifts on the one who cares. We learn to accept ourselves with honesty, patience, and warmth. We fall in love with the beautiful child we once were. We enlarge the boundaries of our heart. Through it we include others in our Self, and we enhance ourselves in the process.

Caring about the well-being of future generations helps us to avoid the pitfalls of the other road, which leads to self-absorption and stagnation. This negative path tempts us into an ever-increasing concern with only ourselves. Persons on this road feel more and more irrelevant as their world and sense

Looking Forward

of self shrink. Eventually despair, meaninglessness, and helplessness dominate daily life and their relations with others.

The good news is that we are given many opportunities to choose the road called generativity. This road beckons us to be newly open in our maturity to places, people, ideas, growth, beauty, dreams, hopes, giving, and rewards. Generativity does not necessarily look peaceful or calm, because all change and growth can be disruptive. Yet when we are living according to this path in a way that is congruent with our inner core, we have chosen the route that will make all the difference in our own lives as well as in those around us.

Health and happiness in our adult years depend on how we see the future and what we do to bring about the kind of future we wish to see. Generativity takes us beyond the short-term gains of daily life and orients us to the long run. What do you imagine when you envision the good that will outlive you?

In this book you have learned to care for yourself in healthy ways, to simplify your life by taking time to reflect and gain insight, to clear away clutter and confusion. You have learned to set limits and have courageously explored both yourself and the conditions around you. You have looked at your spiritual life as it relates to the aging process. You have examined your fears and imagined your future. You have begun to envision a better world for yourself, your friends and your families. You have begun to imagine your future in such a way that you have become sensitized to the sacredness of your life on this Earth.

I once read an African proverb that said, "The world was not left to us by our parents. It was lent to us by our children." What survives you and me are the world's children. I imagine them awaiting our wisdom, wondering how they will embrace their own "next 50 years"—they are innocent and dependent on our ability to share what we have learned. The future looks to each of us with hope.

Dear future generations of women, my wish for you is:

_____

_____

_____

_____

_____

_____

39 Fountain Place

Your black and white marble floors and 4th floor walkup stairs, cool to the touch
concave smoothness now, like some rundown monument
to forgotten immigrants, their accents mingling, reaching out
from acneed ecru walls and crushed, cracked tiles, their
misspelled names engraved in modern walls at Ellis Island.
Generations of bicycles, baby buggies, scooters and carts
have crammed your crud-stung caves in stairwells, damp,
sensuous lovers' kisses given and stolen there.
Stories sung and told in many different tongues
still echoing here, are layered in time, significant
remnants of flapper days, zoot-suit craze and prohibition,
purple haze and prostitution; but in earlier days,
war blackouts, ration stamps, Mayor LaGuardia reading funny papers,
modern plagues and evolution recorded in stone, plaster and lead-based
paint. Iceman, tinker, refugee, bring out your waste to the chanting
junkman, patiently plodding, ringing-bell nodding broken down
sway-back horse and jingly cart up Huguenot Street, wound
around and down North Avenue past the Lutheran Church
and back again like absent-minded clockwork
or an impossible 500-piece jigsaw puzzle on Gramma's card table,
redcoats on horses jumping hedges, hunting foxes, horns trumpeting,
hooves galloping, maidens waving handkerchiefs at the sun.
Tar paper roofs and horses hooves, indelible mind prints.
Even then there were no fountains.
Gramma's place, 4th floor walkup, is still there.
I almost knocked on her door last October, but was afraid to see who might be
living there now,
knowing full well that her lacy curtains fresh from stretching dry on wooden racks,
and her hand-made doilies would be gone,
her dresser drawers so fresh with their soapy scented silky-white
cotton sheets ironed and folded just so,
would not be there anymore.
The bedroom where once I tasted her perfume and spit it out the window,
where I wrote my name in powder on her mirrored dressing table top.
Oriental rug living room floor where we slept on those scented white sheets
on steaming nights with no cross ventilation at all.
Small kitchen where the iceman put the block
and mom fed me pablum so fast that I choked.
Sometimes Gramma smoked a cigarette,
blowing the smoke out that kitchen window.
Where the toaster sat on oilcloth, its angled,
tipping sides always overcooking the bread

so we had to scrape the black off before eating it.
I'm sure a speck of her raspberry jam lies somewhere
on the woodwork beneath 50 coats of paint.
The closet in her room where the monster lived,
bright glowing eyes, may be living among
synthetics now, instead of wool and mothballs.
Deep white tub, wooden tugboats
in a sea of bubbles, her calling,
"don't stand up in the tub until I get there,"
Strauss playing on the radio . . .
Oh, God, how I miss her

—Marilyn Houston

Study Guide

How to Use This Study Guide

This guide is designed to assist book groups in providing a meaningful forum for the discussion of personal experiences and concerns relative to the aging process.

Facilitation: The group may be led by a female professional, or the group members themselves may each take a turn at facilitating. The facilitator must provide a safe and comfortable environment. Be sure to provide tissues, water to drink, and paper cups at each session. She must keep the group on topic as well as assure that each session starts and ends on time. In addition, the facilitator's role is to inform the members how to prepare for the next session. Members are responsible for coming to each session with their own copy of the book, a journal (or notebook), and a pen.

Timing: Each session is designed to last about one and a half to two hours, depending on the size of the group and the weight of the topic. It is suggested that the group meet each week or every other week to create continuity, support, and bonding among the members.

Closing: The closing is the same for each session. While the group stands in a circle holding hands, each member in turn says briefly what she is grateful for in her life.

NOTE: Some topics may lend themselves to two sessions and the facilitator should decide this ahead of time.

Session 1

Goal: Examine and discuss the overall goals for the study group and become acquainted with one another.

Facilitator: Light a candle and assure the group that they are in a safe space where they can speak their hearts and minds without judgment. Name tags are recommended at least for the first session or two. Ask each member in turn to give her first name, age, marital status, whether she has children or not, career or job information, and what she is hoping to get from the study group experience. Write down each woman's goal on a large newsprint pad so the group can see it.

Following the introductions, ask the group to pick three words that describe their personal experience of the aging process. (Facilitator writes these on a clean newsprint page.) Discuss how our aging processes are the same and/or different.

Preparation for the next session: Read the introduction and chapter 1 and write responses to the questions. Be prepared to share a photo of your mother (or other female caregiver) with the group.

Closing

Session 2

Goal: Examine how the cultural attitudes and myths about women and aging affect us.

Facilitator: Ask if anyone in the group is willing to read aloud her written responses to the reading that was assigned in the first session. Ask the group members to share the photos of their mothers.

Questions for discussion (NOTE: the phrase "primary female caregiver" should be used in addition to the word "mother"):

- What positives do you remember about your mother's aging?
- What negatives do you remember about your mother's aging?
- If you didn't have the opportunity to see your mother age (untimely death or other loss), who is your role model for aging?
- What myth about aging would you like to dispel?
- What attitude towards you is most hurtful?

Preparation for the next session: Bring in several magazines, catalogs, or newspapers that show older women in a negative or positive light. Prepare to discuss how the media make us feel about ourselves as aging women. Read chapter 2 and write responses to questions.

Closing

Session 3

Goal: Examine our insights and concerns about our changing bodies and looks.

Facilitator: Ask if anyone in the group is willing to read aloud her written responses to the reading that was assigned in the previous session.

Exercise: Provide glue and scissors and one 11-by-14 piece of cardboard for each member. Have them cut out some of the media images of women they were assigned to bring with them and create a collage on the cardboard. Next have them quietly contemplate what each image is saying to them and write these thoughts in their journal or directly on the collage.

Questions for discussion:

- What do the images on your collage say about aging women?
- Did you have trouble finding positive images of older women that were not detrimental to your self image?

Preparation for the next session: Read chapter 3 and write responses to questions.

Closing

Session 4

Goal: Examine how we view our aging brain and its potential for growth.

Facilitator: Ask if anyone in the group is willing to read aloud her written responses to the reading that was assigned in the previous session.

Questions for discussion:

- Are you aware of any changes in mental capacity?
- What bothers you the most in terms of memory issues?
- How do you see the role of continued learning in your life? Important? Unimportant? What would you like to learn next?

Exercise: On a sheet of blank paper, write two headings:

- Things I have no trouble remembering.
- Things I have trouble remembering.

Notice which list is longer and where you have difficulty. Do you have difficulty remembering relevant or irrelevant information? What does this tell you about yourself or the things you value?

Preparation for the next session: Read chapter 4 and write responses to questions.

Closing

Session 5

Goal: Examine our general emotional response to aging.

Facilitator: Ask if anyone in the group is willing to read aloud her written responses to the reading that was assigned in the previous session.

Questions for discussion:

- What aspect of aging creates an emotional response in you?
- What makes you happy? Mad? Sad?
- How are your emotional responses to life different from when you were younger?
- Do you handle your emotions better or worse now that you're older?

Preparation for the next session: Read chapter 5 and write responses to questions.

Closing

Session 6

Goal: Confront our fears of aging and discuss ways we can overcome them.

Facilitator: Ask if anyone in the group is willing to read aloud her written responses to the reading that was assigned in the previous session.

Questions for discussion:

- What are you most afraid of?
- What are you least afraid of?
- What do you do to cope with your fearful feelings? Do you communicate them?

Preparation for the next session: Search newspapers or magazines for the personal ads section (i.e., men seeking women, women seeking men) and bring the entire newspaper or magazine page with you to the next session. Also, bring in a memento from your love relationship (past or present) that has meaning for you. Read chapter 6 and write responses to questions.

Closing

Session 7

Goal: Consider the role that companionship, love, and sexual expression play in the lives of older women. (Note: These topics may need to be explored in more than one session.)

Facilitator: Ask if anyone in the group is willing to read aloud her written responses to the reading that was assigned in the previous session.

Questions for discussion:

- In the personal ads you were asked to bring with you for this session, what did you notice about what the men were looking for in relationship?
- If you brought in a memento from a past or present relationship, what does it mean to you?
- How are your expectations regarding relationships different from or the same as when you were 30? What is most important now?
- What differences in your sexuality have you experienced? What concerns you the most?

Exercise: Whether you're currently in a relationship or not, write a personal ad for yourself and share it with the group.

Preparation for the next session: Bring a deeply meaningful or spiritually symbolic object with you to share with the group. Read chapter 7 and write responses to questions.

Closing

Session 8

Goal: Examine our spiritual nature and expression as it relates to aging.

Facilitator: Make sure there is a small table placed in the center of the group for the exercise. Light a candle. Ask if anyone in the group is willing to read aloud her written responses to the reading that was assigned in the previous session.

Exercise: The members were asked to bring a meaningful/spiritual object to this session. Ask each group member to place the object on the table in the center of the group and tell what it represents or means to her.

Questions for discussion:

- What brings meaning to your life?
- How do you define spirituality?
- Is spirituality important to you?
- How has your spiritual journey changed over the years?

Preparation for the next session: Read chapter 8 and write responses to questions. Bring with you an example of something you have created and a box of crayons.

Closing

Session 9

Goal: Clarify the role creativity plays in your aging process.

Facilitator: Ask if anyone in the group is willing to read aloud her written responses to the reading that was assigned in the previous session. Invite those who brought in creative projects to "show and tell."

Exercise: Provide 8 1/2-by-11 white paper for each group member. Using crayons, draw a symbol of aging, and with a pen, write a brief paragraph next to or below your drawing describing what this symbol means to you.

Questions for discussion:

- When you expressed a desire to be creative when you were a child, what were you told?
- How do you feel when you've had the opportunity to be creative? Give examples.

Preparation for the next session: Read chapter 9 and write responses to questions.

Closing

Session 10

Goal: Discuss health challenges that affect us as we age.

Facilitator: Ask if anyone in the group is willing to read aloud her written responses to the reading that was assigned in the previous session.

Questions for discussion:

- What was your overall reaction to the chapter on health?
- In what ways have you neglected your health?
- In what ways are you taking care of yourself?
- What are you most concerned about in terms of your health?
- How did your mother or older role model care for herself?

Preparation for the next session: Read chapter 10 and write responses to questions. Do some Internet, magazine, or library research on retirement, adult living, or care facility options that seem desirable to you. Bring your findings to the next session.

Closing

Session 11

Goal: Discuss how we want to live and where we want to live as we age.

Facilitator: Ask if anyone in the group is willing to read aloud her written responses to the reading that was assigned in the previous session.

Questions for discussion:

- What mature adult living choices have you considered?
- Where would you feel most comfortable?
- What situation would be most difficult to adjust to?
- Have you ever visited someone in a facility for the aged? How did you feel?
- Has an elderly relative ever lived with you? Was the experience positive or negative?

Preparation for the next session: Read chapter 11 and write responses to questions. Bring in a photo or two of your current family.

Closing

Session 12

Goal: Discover and discuss the role our families play in our aging experience.

Facilitator: Ask if anyone in the group is willing to read aloud her written responses to the reading that was assigned in the previous session.

Exercise: The members were asked to bring a photo (or photos) of their current family to this session. Each group member in turn holds up or passes around the photo(s) of her family.

Questions for discussion:

- How important is family in your life?
- Do they treat you differently now that you're older?
- What part do you play in your family?
- Has your partner or family expressed how they feel about your aging?
- Have you been teased or made fun of by your family? Do you feel abused or mistreated in any way?

Preparation for the next session: Read chapter 12 and write responses to questions.

Closing

Session 13

Goal: Examine how our friends and community affect our quality of life as we age.

Facilitator: Ask if anyone in the group is willing to read aloud her written responses to the reading that was assigned in the previous session.

Exercise: On a sheet of paper, make eight columns with the following ages: 1–10, 10–20, 20–30, 30–40, 40–50, 50–60, 60–70, 70-plus. Under each heading list the qualities that are (or will be) most important to you in friendship and community as you age.

Questions for discussion:

- Are friends important to you? Why?
- Whom do you feel most comfortable with? Women your own age or younger? Why?
- Do you make time for friends? How?
- Have your expectations for friendship and community changed now that you're older?

Preparation for the next session: Read chapter 13 and write responses to questions. Bring in something (a game, a book, a joke, a creative project, a toy, etc.) that delights the child within you and/or cut a picture out of a magazine that depicts a trip you would like to take or an adventure you would like to experience.

Closing

Session 14

Goal: Discover the energy and benefits that childlike fun, adventure, and curiosity can bring to the aging process.

Facilitator: Ask if anyone in the group is willing to read aloud her written responses to the reading that was assigned in the previous session.

Exercise: The members were asked to bring to this session something (a game, a book, a joke, a creative project, a toy, etc.) that delights the child within and/or a picture that depicts a trip they would like to take or an adventure they would like to have. Each group member in turn holds up or passes around what she brought in.

Questions for discussion:

- Do you have an inner child? If so, what age do you suppose she is?
- Imagine taking your inner child on a vacation. Where would she like to go? Why?
- Imagine going to a movie with your inner child. What would she like to see?
- Your inner child would like to have a play date with you. What would you do?

Preparation for the next session: Read chapter 14 and write responses to questions.

Closing

Session 15

Goal: Examine what work means to us as we age.

Facilitator: Ask if anyone in the group is willing to read aloud her written responses to the reading that was assigned in the previous session.

Questions for discussion:

- Does your definition of work include doing what you love?
- What kind of work (inside or outside the home) have you been engaged in until now?
- What work do you see yourself doing five years from now? Ten years? Twenty years?
- What kind of work would give you the most satisfaction?
- How important is it that you be paid for what you do? Is volunteering an option for you?

Preparation for the next session: Read chapter 15 and write responses to questions.

Closing

Session 16

Goal: Expose and examine our relationship to money and what financial challenges we face as we age.

Facilitator: Ask if anyone in the group is willing to read aloud her written responses to the reading that was assigned in the previous session.

Questions for discussion:

- When you answered the questions in the money section, which one was most difficult to consider? Why?
- How has your relationship to money changed over the years?
- What financial issues concern you the most in the present? In the future?

Preparation for next session: Read chapter 16 and write responses to questions. Bring a photo of yourself as a younger woman (in your twenties or thirties) to the next session.

Closing

Session 17

Goal: Say goodbye to your younger self and then envision the dreams you have for your future and for future generations of women.

Facilitator: Ask if anyone in the group is willing to read aloud her written responses to the reading that was assigned in the previous session. *Discuss responses in depth.*

First Exercise: Place the photo of your younger self in front of you and write a letter to her. Include what she has given you that you will now take into the future, and what she represents that you will need to leave behind to make room for the new you that is emerging.

Second Exercise: Each group member is asked to read aloud her "letter to future generations of women" from the exercise in the book on page 304.

Preparation for the next session: Nothing to prepare.

Closing

Final Session

Goal: The goal of this final session is to have the group members leave with good feelings about themselves and the aging process.

Questions for discussion:

- What exercises or discussions were most valuable to you?
- How have you grown from this group experience?
- What do you want for yourself in the future?

Exercise: Light a candle. Hand out one blank note card and a pen to each member. Invite the women to think quietly about the other group members and then write a wish for each on the card. The facilitator should do this also.

Beginning with the facilitator, read aloud the wish for each member.

A sample card might read:

My wish for you (fill in group member's name):
Alison, is that you overcome your fear of traveling alone.
Margaret, is that you learn to feel comfortable with your body.
Sue, is that you will find a solution to your back pain.
Kathy, is that you learn to take time for yourself.
Jane, is that you overcome your fear of aging.
Debra, is that you enjoy your retirement.

Closing

Bibliography

AARP. *AARP the Magazine.* Washington, D.C.: American Association of Retired Persons.

———. *Think of Your Future: Workbook.* Washington, D.C.: American Association of Retired Persons, 1995.

Alexander, Jo, et al. *Women and Aging: An Anthology by Women.* Corvallis, Ore.: Calyx Books, 1986.

Anderson, Joan. *A Year by the Sea: Thoughts of an Unfinished Woman.* New York: Doubleday, 1999.

Banner, Lois W. *In Full Flower: Aging Women, Power, and Sexuality.* New York: Random House, 1992.

Barnes, Kate. *Where the Deer Were.* Boston, Mass.: David R. Godine, 1994.

Beattie, Melody. *Journey to the Heart: Daily Meditations on the Path to Freeing Your Soul.* San Francisco: HarperSanFrancisco, 1996.

Beckford, Ruth. *Still Groovin': Affirmations for Women in the Second Half of Life.* Naperville, Ill.: Sourcebooks, Inc., 1999.

Bell, Valerie. *A Well-Tended Soul: Staying Beautiful for the Rest of Your Life.* Grand Rapids, Mich.: Zondervan Publishing House, 1996.

———. *She Can Laugh at the Days to Come: Strengthening the Soul for the Journey Ahead.* Grand Rapids, Mich.: Zondervan Publishing House, 1996.

Bender, Sue. *Everyday Sacred: A Woman's Journey Home.* New York: HarperCollins, 1995.

———. *Stretching Lessons: The Daring That Starts from Within.* New York, HarperCollins, 2001.

Biaggi, Christina (ed.). *In the Footsteps of the Goddess: Personal Stories.* Manchester, Conn.: Knowledge, Ideas & Trends, 2000.

Birkedahl, Nonie. *Older and Wiser: A Workbook for Coping with Aging.* Oakland, Calif.: New Harbinger Publications, Inc., 1991.

Black, Cynthia (ed.). *Our Turn, Our Time: Women Truly Coming of Age.* Hillsboro, Ore.: Beyond Words Publishing, 2000.

Bloomfield, Harold. *Making Peace with Your Past: The Six Essential Steps to Enjoying a Great Future.* New York: HarperCollins, 2000.

Bolen, Jean Shinoda. *Crossing to Avalon: A Woman's Midlife Pilgrimage.* New York: HarperCollins, 1994.

Borysenko, Joan. *A Woman's Book of Life: The Biology, Psychology, and Spirituality of the Feminine Life Cycle.* New York: Riverhead Books, 1996.

Bracken, Peg. *On Getting Old for the First Time.* Wilsonville, Ore.: BookPartners, Inc., 1997.

Breathnach, Sarah Ban. *Simple Abundance.* New York: Warner Books, 1995.

Brehony, Kathleen A. *Awakening at Midlife: Realizing Your Potential for Growth and Change.* New York: Riverhead Books, 1996.

Brenner, Marie. *Great Dames: What I Learned from Older Women.* New York: Crown Publishers, 2000.

Brody, Steve, and Cathy Brody. *Renew Your Marriage at Midlife.* New York: Putnam, 1999.

Brooke, Elisabeth. *Medicine Women: A Pictorial History of Women Healers.* Wheaton, Ill.: Godsfield Press/The Theosophical Publishing House/Quest Books, 1997.

Brown, Helen Gurley. *The Late Show: A Semiwild but Practical Survival Plan for Women over 50.* New York: William Morrow & Company, 1993.

Cameron, Julia. *The Artist's Way.* New York: G. P. Putnam's Sons, 1992.

Carson, Lillian. *The Essential Grandparent: A Guide to Making a Difference.* Deerfield Beach, Fla.: Health Communications, 1996.

Cary, Cynthia. *A Foxy Old Woman's Guide to Living with Friends.* Freedom, Calif.: The Crossing Press, 1998.

Chan, Janis Fisher. *Inventing Ourselves Again: Women Face Middle Age.* Portland, Ore.: Sibyl Publications, 1996.

Claflin, Edward (ed.). *Age Protectors: Stop Aging Now.* Emmaus, Pa.: Rodale Press/Prevention Health Books, 1998.

Claman, Elizabeth (ed.). *Each in Her Own Way: Women Writing on the Menopause.* Eugene, Ore.: Queen of Sword Press, 1994.

Cleveland, Joan. *Simplifying Life as a Senior Citizen.* New York: St. Martin's Press, 1998.

Clinebell, Howard. *Well Being: A Personal Plan for Exploring and Enriching the Seven Dimensions of Life.* San Francisco: HarperSanFrancisco, 1992.

Cohen, Gene D. *The Creative Age: Awakening Human Potential in the Second Half of Life.* New York: Avon Books, 2000.

Cohen, Leah. *Small Expectations: Society's Betrayal of Older Women.* Toronto, Canada: McClelland and Stewart, 1984.

Crenshaw, Theresa. *The Alchemy of Love and Lust.* New York: G. P. Putnam's Sons, 1996.

Crisp, Wendy Reid. *100 Things I'm Not Going to Do Now That I'm over 50.* New York: Berkley Publishing Group, 1995.

Crowe, Sandra. *Since Strangling Isn't an Option: Dealing with Difficult People.* New York: Perigee Book, 1999.

Dailey, Nancy. *When Baby Boom Women Retire.* Westport, Conn.: Praeger Publishers, 2000.

Davis, Nancy D., et al. (eds.). *Faces of Women and Aging.* New York: Haworth Press, 1993.

Dean, Amy E. *Night Light.* Center City, Minn.: Hazelden, 1986.

———. *Growing Older, Growing Better: Daily Meditations for Celebrating Aging.* Carlsbad, Calif.: Hay House, Inc., 1997.

de Castillejo, Irene Claremont. *Knowing Woman: A Feminine Psychology.* Boston, Mass.: Shambhala, 1997.

Delany, Sarah L. *On My Own at 107: Reflections on Life without Bessie.* New York: HarperSanFrancisco, 1997.

Delany, Sarah L., and A. Elizabeth Delany. *Having Our Say: The Delaney Sisters' First 100 Years.* Thorndike, Maine: G.K. Hall, 1993.

Diekemper, Lou Dunn. *Women Who Take Care. Choosing to Live with Wisdom, Grace, and Power after Fifty-Five!* Nevada City, Calif.: Blue Dolphin Publishing, 1997.

Doherty, Dorothy Albracht, and Mary Colgan McNamara. *Out of the Skin into the Soul: The Art of Aging.* San Diego, Calif.: LuraMedia, 1993.

Dollemore, Doug, et al. *Seniors Guide to Pain-Free Living.* Emmaus, Pa.: Rodale, Inc., 2000.

Doress-Worters, Paula B., and Diana Laskin Siegal. *The New Ourselves, Growing Older: Women Aging with Knowledge and Power.* New York: Touchstone, 1994.

Dowling, Colette. *Red Hot Mamas.* New York: Bantam Books, 1996.

Downes, Peggy, et al. *The New Older Woman: A Dialogue for the Coming Century.* Berkeley, Calif.: Celestial Arts, 1996.

Ealy, C. Diane. *The Woman's Book of Creativity.* Hillsboro, Ore.: Beyond Words Publishing, 1995.

Eckford, Leslie, and Amanda Lambert. *Beating the Senior Blues: How to Feel Better and Enjoy Life Again.* Oakland, Calif.: New Harbinger Publications, 2002.

Eisler, Riane. *The Chalice and the Blade: Our History, Our Future.* Cambridge, Mass.: Harper & Row, 1987.

Ellis, Neenah. *If I Live to Be 100: Lessons from the Centenarians.* New York: Crown Publishers, 2002.

Ellison, Carol Rinkleib. *Women's Sexualities: Generations of Women Share Intimate Secrets of Sexual Self-Acceptance.* Oakland, Calif.: New Harbinger Publications, 2000.

Feldman, Susan, et al. *Something That Happens to Other People: Stories of Women Growing Older.* New York: Vintage, 1996.

Field, Joanna. *A Life of One's Own.* London: Virago, 1986.

Finn, Susan Calvert. *Women's Nutrition for Healthy Living.* New York: Berkley Publishing Group, 1997.

Fisher, M. F. K. *Sister Age.* New York: Alfred A. Knopf, 1983.

Frank, Joan. *Desperate Women Need to Talk to You.* Emeryville, Calif.: Conari Press, 1994.

Freeman, Phyllis R., and Jan Zlotnik Schmidt. *Wise Women.* New York: Routledge, 2000.

Friday, Nancy. *The Power of Beauty.* London: Hutchinson, 1996.

Friedan, Betty. *The Fountain of Age.* New York: Simon & Schuster, 1993.

———. *Life So Far.* New York: Touchstone, 2000.

Furman, Frida Kerner. *Facing the Mirror: Older Women and Beauty Shop Culture.* New York and London: Routledge, 1997.

Gendler, J. Ruth. *The Book of Qualities.* New York: Harper & Row, 1988.

Gerzon, Mark. *Listening to Midlife: Turning Your Crisis into a Quest.* Boston, Mass.: Shambhala, 1992.

Godwin, Gail. *Evenings at Five.* New York: Ballantine Books, 2003.

Goldberg, Natalie. *Long Quiet Highway: Waking Up in America.* New York: Bantam Books, 1993.

Goldman, Connie, and Richard Mahler. *Secrets of Becoming a Late Bloomer.* Walpole, N.H.: Stillpoint, 1995.

Goodwin, Gail. *Fabulous Friends: A Celebration of Girlfriendship.* Kansas City, Mo.: Andrews McMeel, 2004.

Gordon, Helen Heightsman. *Age Is a Laughing Matter: How to Laugh through the Second Half of Your Life.* Santa Barbara, Calif.: Anacade International, 1999.

Grafton, Sue (ed.). *Writing Mysteries: A Handbook*. Cincinnati, Ohio: Writer's Digest Books, 1992.

Greene, Phyllis. *Shedding Years: Growing Older, Feeling Younger*. New York: Villard, 2003.

Gross, Zenith Henkin. *Season of the Heart: Men and Women Talk about Love, Sex, and Romance after 60*. Novato, Calif.: New World Library, 2000.

Grumbach, Doris. *Fifty Days of Solitude*. Boston, Mass.: Beacon Press, 1994.

Harper, Valerie. *Today I Am a Ma'am: And Other Musings on Life, Beauty, and Growing Older*. New York: Cliff Street Books, 2001.

Hauser, Susan Carol. *Full Moon: Reflections on Turning Fifty*. Watsonville, Calif.: Papier-Mache Press, 1996.

Hay, Louise L. *Heal Your Body: Journey to the Heart*. New York: HarperCollins, 1996.

Hayes, Helen, with Marion Glasserow Gladney. *Helen Hayes*. New York: Doubleday & Co., 1984.

Haynes, Marion E. *PrimeLife Guide to Personal Success: A Planning Guide for the 40-Plus Generation*. Menlo Park, Calif.: Crisp Publications, 1996.

Hazard, Claudia, and Hears Crow. *She Is Beautiful*. Owings Mills, Md.: Watermark Press, 1996.

Heffler, Ira, and Jerry Schneider. *How to Create a Video Biography: A Legacy for Your Family*. Carlsbad, Calif.: Arrowhead Publishing, 1999.

Heilbrun, Carolyn G. *The Last Gift of Time: Life beyond Sixty*. New York: Ballantine Books, 1997.

Heilman, Joan Rattner. *Unbelievably Good Deals and Great Adventures That You Absolutely Can't Get unless You're over 50, 2005–2006*. Chicago, Ill.: Contemporary Books/McGraw Hill, 2004.

Hemmings, Susan (ed.). *A Wealth of Experience: The Lives of Older Women*. London and Boston: Pandora Press, 1985.

Hen Co-Op, The. *Disgracefully Yours: More New Ideas for Getting the Most Out of Life*. Freedom, Calif.: Crossing Press, 1996.

Henderson, Sallirae. *A Life Complete: Finding Peace and Purpose at Midlife*. New York: Fireside/Simon & Schuster, 2000.

Holland, Barbara. *One's Company: Reflections on Living Alone*. New York: Ballantine Books, 1992.

———. *Wasn't the Grass Greener?: A Curmudgeon's Fond Memories*. New York: Harcourt Brace, 1999.

Hossack, Joei Carlton. *A Million Miles from Home*. Sarasota, Fla.: Skeena Press, 2002.

Jacobs, Ruth Harriet. *Be an Outrageous Older Woman*. New York: Harper Perennial/HarperCollins Publishers, 1997.

Jarvis, Cheryl. *The Marriage Sabbatical: The Journey That Brings You Home*. Cambridge, Mass.: Perseus Publishing, 2001.

Johnson, Barbara. *Living Somewhere between Estrogen and Death*. Dallas, Tex.: Word Publishing, 1997.

Kaigler-Walker, Karen. *Positive Aging: Every Woman's Quest for Wisdom and Beauty*. Berkeley, Calif.: Conari Press, 1997.

Katz, Lawrence C., and Manning Rubin. *Keep Your Brain Alive*. New York: Workman Pub., 1999.

Kingsolver, Barbara. *Pigs in Heaven*. New York: HarperPerennial, 1994.

Kitzinger, Sheila. *Becoming a Grandmother: A Life Transition*. London: Pocket Books/Simon & Schuster, 1997.

Krantzler, Mel. *Learning to Love Again*. New York: Crowell, 1977.

Latimer, Rebecca. *You're Not Old until You're Ninety*. Nevada City, Calif.: Blue Dolphin Publishing, 1997.

Ledoux, Denis. *Turning Memories into Memoirs*. Lisbon Falls, Maine: Soleil Press, 1993.

L'Engle, Madeleine. *A Circle of Quiet*. New York: Farrar, Straus and Giroux, 1972.

——. *The Irrational Season*. New York: Seabury Press, 1977.

LeShan, Eda. *Oh, to Be 50 Again! It's the Time of Your Life—Make the Most of It Now!* New York: Pocket Books, 1986.

——. *It's Better to Be over the Hill Than under It*. New York: Newmarket Press, 1990.

Lesnoff-Caravaglia, Gari (ed.). *The World of the Older Woman: Conflicts and Resolutions*. New York: Human Science Press, 1984.

Lindbergh, Anne Morrow. *Gift from the Sea*. New York: Random House, 1997.

Lindquist, Marie. *Holding Back*. New York: Harper & Row, 1988.

MacLaine, Shirley. *Going Within: A Guide for Inner Transformation*. New York: Bantam Books, 1989.

Maisel, Eric. *Affirmations for Artists*. New York: Penguin Putnam, Inc., 1996.

Marston, Stephanie. *If Not Now, When? Reclaiming Ourselves at Midlife*. New York: Warner Books, 2001.

Martindale, Judith A., and Mary J. Moses. *Creating Your Own Future: A Woman's Guide to Retirement Planning*. Naperville, Ill.: Sourcebooks Trade, 1991.

Martz, Sandra Haldeman (ed.). *Grow Old Along with Me, the Best Is Yet to Be.* Watsonville, Calif.: Papier-Mache Press, 1996.

McCall, Edith. *Sometimes We Dance Alone: Your Next Years Can Be Your Best Years!* Brooklyn, N.Y.: Brett Books, Inc., 1994.

McConnell, Mary. *Still Dancing: Life Choices and Challenges for Women.* Tucson, Ariz.: Harbinger House, Inc., 1990.

McLeod, Beth Witrogen (ed.). *And Thou Shalt Honor: The Caregiver's Companion.* Emmaus, Pa.: Rodale, 2002.

McWade, Micki. *Getting Up, Getting Over, Getting On: A Twelve Step Guide to Divorce Recovery.* Fredonia, Wis.: Champion Press, 1999.

———. *Daily Meditations for Surviving a Breakup, Separation, or Divorce* (Getting Up, Getting Over, Getting on Series). Fredonia, Wis.: Champion Press, 2002.

Melamed, Elissa. *Mirror Mirror: The Terror of Not Being Young.* New York: Linden Press/Simon & Schuster, 1983.

Mitchell, Shirley, and Jane Rubietta. *Fabulous after 50: Finding Fulfillment for Tomorrow.* Green Forest, Ariz.: New Leaf Press, 2000.

Moffatt, BettyClare. *Soulwork: Clearing the Mind, Opening the Heart, Replenishing the Spirit.* Berkeley, Calif.: Wildcat Canyon Press, 1994.

———. *An Authentic Woman: Soulwork for the Wisdom Years.* New York: Simon & Schuster, 1999.

Morris, Monica. *Looking for Love in Later Life: A Woman's Guide to Finding Joy and Romantic Fulfillment.* Garden City Park, N.Y.: Avery Publishing Group, 1997.

Morrissey, Lynn D. (ed.). *Seasons of a Woman's Heart: A Daybook of Stories and Inspiration.* Lancaster, Pa.: Starburst Publishers, 1999.

Morrison, Mary C. *Without Nightfall upon the Spirit.* Wallingford, Pa.: Pendle Hill Publications, 1994.

———. *Let Evening Come: Reflections on Aging.* New York: Doubleday, 1998.

Murdock, Maureen. *The Heroine's Journey Workbook.* Boston, Mass.: Shambhala, 1998.

Nearing, Helen. *Wise Words for the Good Life.* White River Junction, Vt.: Chelsea Green Pub., 1999.

Nickerson, Betty. *Old and Smart: Women and Aging.* Eugene, Ore.: All About Us Books, 1991.

Noel, Brook, and Pamela Blair. *I Wasn't Ready to Say Goodbye: Surviving, Coping, and Healing after the Sudden Death of a Loved One.* Milwaukee, Wis.: Champion Press, 2000.

Norman, Marsha. *The Fortune Teller*. New York: Random House, 1989.

Northrup, Christiane. *Women's Bodies, Women's Wisdom: Creating Physical and Emotional Health and Healing*. New York: Bantam Books, 1998.

——. *Health Wisdom for Women* newsletter. Potomac, Md.: Phillips Publishing (various dates).

Norwood, Robin. *Women Who Love Too Much: When You Keep Wishing and Hoping He'll Change*. Los Angeles: J. P. Tarcher, 1985.

Nudel, Adele. *For the Woman over 50: A Practical Guide for a Full and Vital Life*. New York: Taplinger Publishing Company, 1978.

Oliver, Mary. *The Leaf and the Cloud*. Cambridge, Mass.: DaCapo Press, 2000.

Orman, Suze. *The 9 Steps to Financial Freedom: Practical and Spiritual Steps so You Can Stop Worrying*. New York: Crown Publishers, 1997.

Pederson, Rena, with Lee Smith. *What's Next?: Women Redefining Their Dreams in the Prime of Life*. New York: Perigee Books/Berkley Publishing/Penguin Putnam, 2001.

Peirce, Penney. *The Present Moment: A Daybook of Clarity and Intuition*. Lincolnwood, Ill.: Contemporary Books/NTC, 2000.

Perls, Thomas T., and Margery Hutter Silver, with John F. Lauerman. *Living to 100: Lessons in Living to Your Maximum Potential at Any Age*. New York: Basic Books/Perseus Books Group, 1999.

Perry, Susan K. *Writing in Flow: Keys to Enhanced Creativity*. Cincinnati, Ohio: Writer's Digest Books, 1999.

Piercy, Marge. *The Moon Is Always Female*. New York: Alfred A. Knopf, 1996.

Pipher, Mary. *Another Country: Navigating the Emotional Terrain of Our Elders*. New York: Riverhead Books/Penguin Putnam, 1999.

Pogrebin, Letty Cottin. *Getting Over Getting Older: An Intimate Journey*. New York: Penguin Putnam, 1992.

Popcorn, Faith, and Adam Hanft. *Dictionary of the Future*. New York: Hyperion, 2001.

Porcino, Jane. *Growing Older, Getting Better: A Handbook for Women in the Second Half of Life*. Reading, Mass.: Addison-Wesley Publishing Company, 1983.

Quinn, Janet F. *I Am a Woman Finding My Voice: Celebrating the Extraordinary Blessings of Being a Woman*. New York: Eagle Brook/William Morrow, 1999.

Reed, Terence L. *The 8 Biggest Mistakes People Make with Their Finances before and after Retirement*. Chicago: Dearborn Trade Publishing, 2001.

Reilly, Patricia Lynn. *Imagine a Woman in Love with Herself: Embracing Your Wisdom and Wholeness*. Berkeley, Calif.: Conari Press, 1999.

The Next Fifty Years

Rivers, Joan. *Don't Count the Candles: Just Keep the Fire Lit.* New York, HarperCollins, 1999.

Robin, Vicki, and Joe Dominguez. *Your Money or Your Life: Transforming Your Relationship with Money and Achieving Financial Independence.* New York: Penguin Books, 1999.

Rountree, Cathleen. *On Women Turning 50: Celebrating Mid-Life Discoveries.* New York: HarperCollins, 1993.

———. *On Women Turning 60: Embracing the Age of Fulfillment.* New York: Harmony Book/Crown, 1997.

———. *On Women Turning 70: Honoring the Voices of Wisdom.* San Francisco, Calif.: Jossey-Bass Publishers, 1999.

———. *The Writer's Mentor: A Guide to Putting Passion on Paper.* Berkeley, Calif.: Conari Press, 2002.

Rowe, John W., and Robert L. Kahn. *Successful Aging.* New York: Dell Publishing, 1998.

Rubin, Bonnie Miller. *Fifty on Fifty: Wisdom, Inspiration, and Reflections on Women's Lives Well Lived.* New York: Warner Books, 1998.

Rupp, Joyce. *Dear Heart, Come Home: The Path of Midlife Spirituality.* New York: Crossroad Publishing, 1996.

Russ, Lavinia. *A High Old Time: Or How to Enjoy Being a Woman over Sixty.* Boston, Mass.: G. K. Hall, 1972.

Russell, Roberta, with R. D. Laing. *R. D. Laing and Me: Lessons in Love.* Lake Placid, N. Y.: Hillgarth Press, 1992.

Sachs, Judith. *Sensual Rejuvenation: Maintaining Sexual Vigor through Midlife and Beyond.* New York: Dell Publishing, 1999.

Sark. *Succulent Wild Woman: Dancing with Your Wonder-full Self!* New York: Fireside/ Simon & Schuster, 1997.

Sarton, May. *Journal of a Solitude.* New York: W. W. Norton & Company, 1973.

———. *At Seventy: A Journal.* New York: W. W. Norton & Company, 1984.

———. *After the Stroke: A Journal.* New York/London: W. W. Norton & Company, 1988.

———. *Endgame: A Journal of the Seventy-Ninth Year.* New York/London: W. W. Norton & Company, 1992.

———. *At Eighty-Two: A Journal.* New York/London: W. W. Norton & Company, 1996.

Savitz, Harriet May. *Growing Up at 62: A Celebration.* Atlantic Highlands, N.J.: Little Treasure Publications, Inc., 1997.

Scarf, Maggie. *Unfinished Business: Pressure Points in the Lives of Women.* New York: Ballantine Books, 1980.

Schacter-Shalomi, Zalman, and Ronald S. Miller. *From Age-ing to Sage-ing: A Profound New Vision of Growing Older.* New York: Warner Books, 1995.

Schlehofer, Jo. *Celebrate the Older You: Becoming a Wiser, Warmer, Mature Woman.* Notre Dame, Ind.: Ave Maria Press, Inc., 1998.

Scott, Lucy. *Wise Choices beyond Midlife: Women Mapping the Journey Ahead.* Watsonville, Calif.: Papier-Mache Press, 1997.

Scott-Maxwell, Florida. *The Measure of My Days.* New York: Penguin Books, 1968.

Shaevitz, Marjorie Hansen. *The Confident Woman: Learn the Rules of the Game.* New York: Harmony Books, 1999.

Sheehy, Gail. *New Passages: Mapping Your Life across Time.* New York: Ballantine Books, 1995.

Sheindlin, Judy (Judge Judy). *Keep It Simple, Stupid: You're Smarter than You Look.* New York: Cliff Street Books, 2000.

Sher, Barbara. *It's Only Too Late if You Don't Start Now: How to Create Your Second Life after 40.* New York: Delacorte Press, 1992.

Simpson, Eileen. *Late Love: A Celebration of Marriage after Fifty.* New York: Houghton Mifflin Company, 1994.

Sinetar, Marsha. *Don't Call Me Old—I'm Just Awakening! Spiritual Encouragement for Later Life.* Mahway, N.J.: Paulist Press, 2002.

Smith, Patricia "Poppy." *I'm Too Young to Be This Old!* Minneapolis, Minn.: Bethany House Publishers, 1997.

Smith, Sarah. *Mid-Life: Coming Home.* Shippensburg, Pa.: Ragged Edge Press, 1999.

Snow, Kimberly. *Word Play Word Power: A Woman's Personal Growth Workbook.* Berkeley, Calif.: Conari Press, 1989.

Start, Clarissa. *I'm Glad I'm Not Young Anymore.* St. Louis, Mo.: The Patrice Press, 1990.

Stasi, Linda, and Rosemary Rogers. *Boomer Babes: A Woman's Guide to the New Middle Ages.* New York: St. Martin's Press, 1998.

Stern, Ellen Sue. *In My Prime: Meditations for Women in Midlife.* New York: Dell Publishing, 1995.

Stewart, Susan, with Sona Dimidjian. *Flying Solo: Single Women in Midlife.* New York: W. W. Norton & Company, 1994.

St. James, Elaine. *Simplify Your Life: 100 Ways to Slow Down and Enjoy the Things That Really Matter.* New York: Hyperion, 1994.

The Next Fifty Years

Stoddard, Alexandra. *Living a Beautiful Life: Five Hundred Ways to Add Elegance, Order, Beauty, and Joy to Every Day of Your Life.* New York: Random House, 1986.

——. *The Art of the Possible.* New York: Avon Books, 1995.

Sumner, Fran. *The Love Affair of Fran and Maurie.* Menlo Park, Calif.: Group Fore Productions, 1997.

Sunila, Joyce. *The New Lovers: Younger Men/Older Women: Wonderful Love Options for Women of All Ages.* New York: Fawcett Gold Medal/Ballantine Books, 1980.

Swallow, Wendy. *Breaking Apart: A Memoir of Divorce.* New York: Hyperion, 2001.

Swartz, Susan. *Juicy Tomatoes: Plain Truths, Dumb Lies, and Sisterly Advice about Life after 50.* Oakland, Calif.: New Harbinger Publications, 2000.

Szynski, Jill A., and Herb I. Kavet. *Women over 50 Are Better Because . . .* Watertown, Mass.: Boston America Corp., 1997.

Taylor, Allegra. *Older Than Time: A Grandmother's Search for Wisdom.* New York: HarperCollins, 1994.

Taylor, Russell R. *Exceptional Entrepreneurial Women.* New York: Praeger Publishers, 1988.

Tenneson, Joyce. *Wise Women: A Celebration of Their Insights, Courage, and Beauty.* Boston: Bulfinch Press/Little, Brown and Company, 2002.

Thoele, Sue Patton. *Freedoms after 50.* Berkeley, Calif. Conari Press, 1998.

Thone, Ruth Raymond. *Women and Aging: Celebrating Ourselves.* Binghamton, N.Y.: Harrington Park Press/Haworth Press, 1992.

Troll, Lillian E., et al. (eds.). *Looking Ahead: A Woman's Guide to the Problems and Joys of Growing Older.* Englewood Cliffs, N.J.: Prentice-Hall, 1977.

Turk, Ruth. *The Second Flowering.* Clinton, N.J.: New Win Publishing, 1993.

Ueland, Brenda. *If You Want to Write.* St. Paul, Minn.: Graywolf Press, 1987.

Vaughn, Ruth, and Anita Higman. *Who Will I Be for the Rest of My Life: Heart to Heart Wisdom for Seasons of Change.* Minneapolis, Minn.: Bethany House Publishers, 1998.

Vickers, Joanne F., and Barbara L. Thomas (interviewers). *No More Frogs, No More Princes: Woman Making Creative Choices at Midlife.* Freedom, Calif.: The Crossing Press, 1993.

Vienne, Veronique. *The Art of Growing Up: Simple Ways to Be Yourself at Last.* New York: Clarkson Potter/Crown, 2000.

Viorst, Judith. *Necessary Losses.* New York: Simon & Schuster, 1986.

——. *Forever Fifty.* New York: Simon & Schuster, 1989.

——. *Suddenly Sixty and Other Shocks of Later Life*. New York: Simon & Schuster, 2000.

Waitley, Denis, and Eudora Seyfer. *How to Be Happily Retired*. Berkeley, Calif.: Celestial Arts, 1995.

Walford, Roy L. *Beyond the 120-Year Diet: How to Double Your Vital Years*. New York: Four Walls Eight Windows, 2000.

Walker, Barbara G. *The Woman's Encyclopedia of Myths and Secrets*. New York: HarperSanFrancisco/HarperCollins, 1983.

Weaver, Frances, *The Girls with the Grandmother Faces*. New York: Hyperion, 1996.

——. *I'm Not as Old as I Used to Be: Reclaiming Your Life in the Second Half*. New York: Hyperion, 1997.

Welch, Elizabeth. *Learning to Be 85*. Nashville, Tenn.: Upper Room Books, 1991.

Wells, Rebecca. *Divine Secrets of the Ya-Ya Sisterhood*. Rockland, Md.: Wheeler Pub., 1998.

West, V. Sackville. *All Passion Spent*. Garden City, N.Y.: Dial Press, 1984.

Wharton, Edith. *A Backward Glance*. New York: Scribner, 1934.

Wiebe, Katie Funk. *Border Crossing: A Spiritual Journey*. Scottsdale, Pa.: Herald Press, 1995.

Williamson, Marianne. *A Woman's Worth*. New York: Random House, 1993.

Wolf, Naomi. *The Beauty Myth: How Images of Beauty Are Used against Women*. New York: Anchor Books/Doubleday/Bantam Doubleday Dell, 1991.

Wyse, Lois. *Funny, You Don't Look Like a Grandmother*. New York: Crown Publishers, 1989.

——. *Women Make the Best Friends*. New York: Simon & Schuster, 1995.

Zielinski, Lynne. *Chocolate for a Woman's Spirit*. New York: Fireside Books, Simon & Schuster, 1999.

Zukerman, Rachelle. *Young at Heart: The Mature Woman's Guide to Finding and Keeping Romance*. New York: Contemporary Books/ McGraw-Hill, 2001.

About the Author

Pamela D. Blair, Ph.D., is a holistic psychotherapist, spiritual counselor, and personal coach with a private practice.

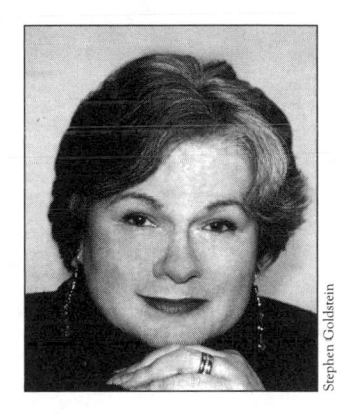

Stephen Goldstein

A frequently invited guest on TV, cable, and radio talk shows, Dr. Blair has appeared several times as an expert on CBS TV and was a regular columnist for *Single Living*, a writer for *American Woman*, and publisher of *Surviving Divorce*. She is currently a contributor to *LifeSherpa Magazine*, *GriefNet.com*, *Divorce Magazine*, *Single Parents Magazine*, and *50+ Magazine*. She is coauthor of the best-selling book on grief entitled *I Wasn't Ready to Say Goodbye* (Champion Press, March 2000) as well as the recently published companion workbook.

Dr. Blair is on the faculty of Wainwright House, Rye, New York, a prestigious facility where she coordinated the Institute for Spiritual Development for four years. Among other places, she has taught at the New York Open Center and the Interface Institute in Massachusetts. Dr. Blair is a member of American Psychotherapy Association, AIM (Association of Interfaith Ministers), the International Women Writers Guild, and the Westchester Holistic Practitioners Network and is the founder of Westchester Women Writers and a Circle of Women, an ongoing therapy group specializing in women at midlife and beyond. She is an Interfaith Minister with a masters from The New Seminary in New York, New York.

Dr. Blair earned her Ph.D. from the American Institute of Holistic Theology in Birmingham, Alabama; has certificates in Integrative Therapy, Therapeutic Touch, and Treating Survivors of Destructive Families; and is a Certified Hospice Counselor. In addition, she studied at the Transformational Training Institute and the New England Educational Institute for Mental Health.

Dr. Blair has three grown children and five grandchildren. She lives in Hawthorne, New York, with her husband, Steve, and two cats.

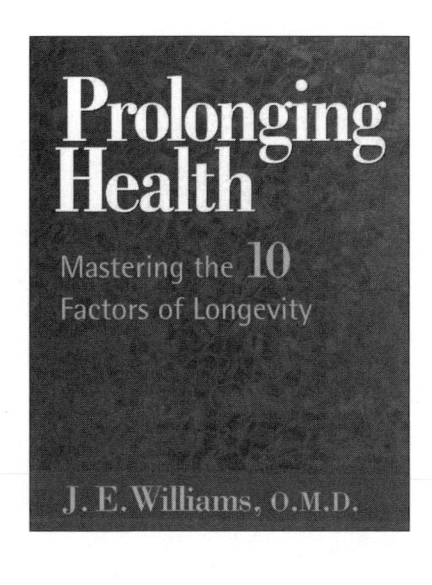

Prolonging Health
Mastering the 10 Factors of Longevity
J. E. Williams, O.M.D.

Aging doesn't have to mean failing physical health, declining mental acuity, disease, frailty, and life in a nursing home. You can extend your good health as you grow older by using the best of natural medicine. In *Prolonging Health,* James Williams, O.M.D. shows that there's no reason you can't live to well over 100 years—enjoying good health all the while.

Based on the latest medical findings, Dr. Williams presents a practical, 10-point plan to prolong your health by understanding and changing the ten major causes of aging. He shows how to strengthen your heart, revitalize your brain, rebalance your hormones, repair your DNA, prevent degenerative disease, detoxify your cells, avoid insulin resistance, and more. He says, "One thing is certain: the better your health, the longer you will live—and live well."

Paperback • 464 pages • ISBN 978-1-57174-338-1 • $17.95

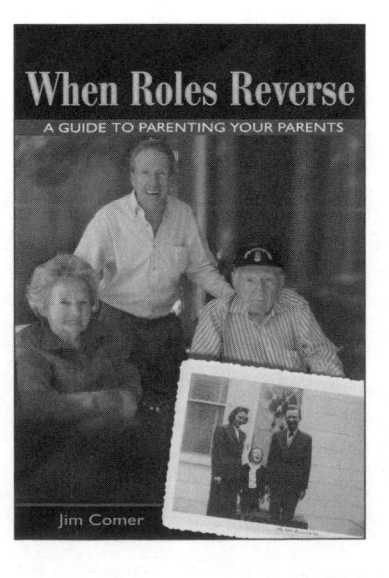

When Roles Reverse
A Guide to Parenting Your Parents
Jim Comer

When his father suffered a massive stroke while caring for his mother who had Alzheimer's, Jim Comer found himself learning to deal with hospitals, insurance companies, rehab centers, Dad's deafness, and Mother's dementia. Combining wit, warmth, and practical advice, *When Roles Reverse* helps families break through denial to initiate the conversations that "will save you time, money, and tears." With laugh-out-loud humor, Comer deals with moments for which there are no preparation and offers personal experience and expert insight on the many issues for which it's absolutely essential to plan.

Paperback • 328 pages • ISBN 978-1-57174-500-2 • $17.95

The Healthy Living Space
70 Practical Ways to Detoxify the Body and Home
Richard Leviton

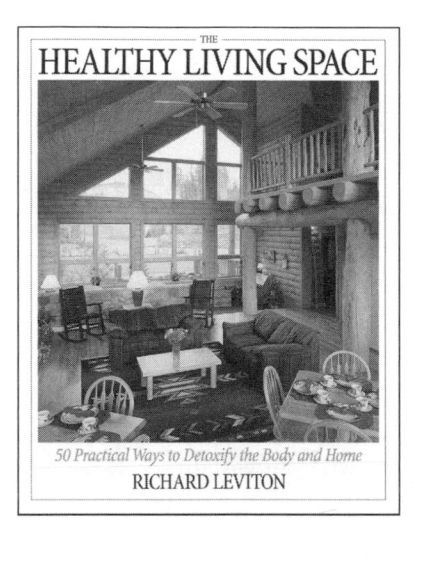

Science shows that nearly every corner of our planet is toxic, and that all people carry residues of dozens of chemicals in their cells. Our body, our home, and our world are steadily sickening us every day of our lives. But we don't have to live in a poisoned world, and we don't have to be sick. We can have a healthy living space again by detoxifying our body and home, ridding both of their toxic burden. The key is to cleanse both at the same time. *The Healthy Living Space* is the first book that shows you how—and why—to detoxify your home and body together. Backed by science and easy to use, the methods of detoxification, drawn from the fields of natural and alternative medicine, don't require expensive equipment or a doctor's supervision. They're effective and produce results and you can start them today.

Paperback • 656 pages • ISBN 978-1-57174-209-4 • $21.95

How People Heal
Exploring the Scientific Basis of Subtle Energy in Healing
Diane Goldner

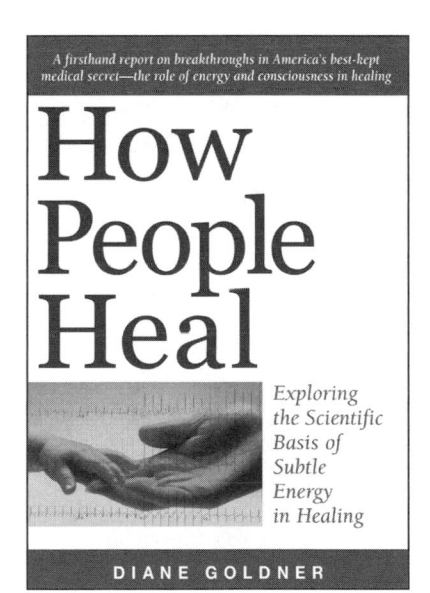

If you've ever gone to an energy healer or been curious about the process, this paperback reissue of Goldner's *Infinite Grace* is for you. Goldner goes in-depth with renowned healers including Barbara Brennan and Rosalyn Bruyere as well as the patients who use energy medicine to positive effect against everything from cancer to AIDS.

How People Heal also introduces you to physicists mapping the effects of love and desire across time and space, nurses using therapeutic touch on hospital patients, and heart surgeons using energy medicine in the operating room. Most importantly, you'll meet people whose lives and life-threatening illnesses have been transformed by the work of energy healers.

Paperback • 360 pages • ISBN 978-1-57174-363-3 • $14.95

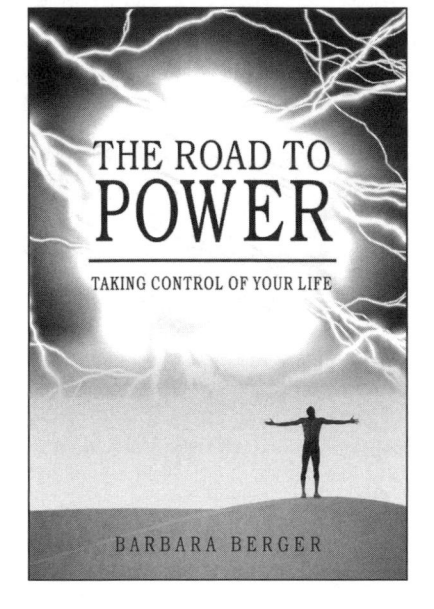

The Road to Power
Taking Control of Your Life

Barbara Berger

In this highly practical book, Berger offers the tools and then guides you step by step into how you can change your life by changing your thinking. If your life is not working, or you just want it to work better, here's a simple yet effective way to look inside yourself and see what you can do about money, relationships, love, your health, family, work, peace, joy, and much more. And it will be faster and easier than you ever dreamed possible.

Paperback • 208 pages • ISBN 978-1-57174-443-2 • $14.95

In 2000 Hampton Roads published Lynn Grabhorn's *Excuse Me, Your Life Is Waiting,* which became a *New York Times* bestseller. Hundreds of thousands of readers have felt their lives transformed by Lynn's message. Lynn's book has brought us positive energy that has attracted other authors whose lives are guided by the principles she espoused. Hampton Roads now offers the following books in the *Excuse Me* series:

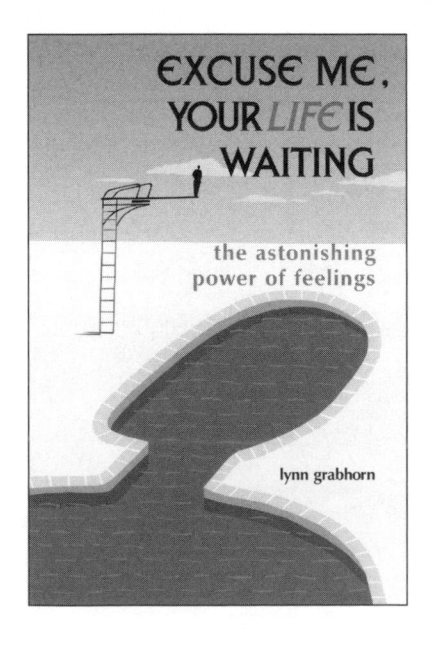

Excuse Me, Your Life Is Waiting
The Astonishing Power of Feelings

Lynn Grabhorn

Ready to get what you want? Half a million readers have answered with an enthusiastic "yes" and have embraced Lynn's principles for achieving the life of their dreams. This upbeat yet down-to-earth book reveals how our true feelings work to "magnetize" and create the reality we experience. Part coach, part cheerleader, Lynn lays out the nuts and bolts of harnessing the raw power of your feelings. Once you become aware of what you're feeling, you'll turn the negatives into positives and literally draw all those good things to you like a magnet, creating the life you know you were meant to have—right now!

Discover the secrets that have made *Excuse Me* a *New York Times* bestseller!

Paperback • 328 pages • ISBN 978-1-57174-381-7 • $16.95

The Excuse Me, Your Life Is Waiting *Playbook*

With the Twelve Tenets of Awakening

Lynn Grabhorn

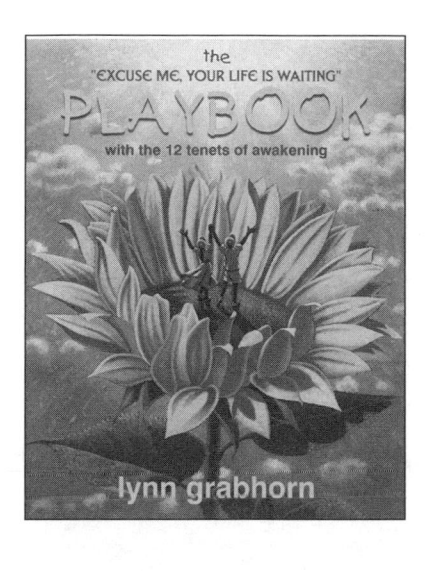

Human beings have evolved physically, socially, and technologically, but are unable to take the next step toward spiritual evolution because of self-defeating habits and conditioning—in short, we are our own victims. Lynn Grabhorn has taken the concepts that made *Excuse Me, Your Life Is Waiting* a bestseller and transformed them into a complete workbook for empowerment. The clearly focused explanations, discussion material, meditations, and exercises are essential building blocks to a new way of being.

Trade paper • 288 pages • ISBN 978-1-57174-270-4 • $22.95

Excuse Me, Your Job Is Waiting

Attract the Work You Want

Laura George

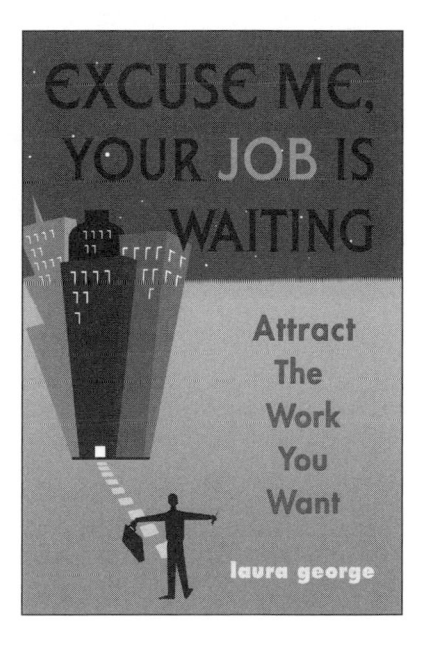

New York Times bestseller author Lynn Grabhorn showed half a million readers how to "magnetize" their emotions to draw their desires to them. Now, human resource manager Laura George applies Grabhorn's powerful Law of Attraction to the life experiences of both losing and getting a job. George captures the style and substance of *Excuse Me* and helps you identify the qualities you want in a job and then shows you how to flip the negative feelings you may be carrying ("the economy is terrible"; "I can't believe I got laid off"; "I'm too old") so you can stay focused and upbeat to draw that perfect job to you.

Experienced in job hunting from both sides of the interview table, George understands all the highs and lows in this emotionally draining process. As a job seeker, she teaches you to stay positive after months of few prospects and little hope. As a human resource manager she also knows that these powerful, positive feelings can land seekers the job of their dreams. By exploring the "power of feelings" on your job search, this new job seeker's guide is unlike any other.

Paperback • 312 pages • ISBN 978-1-57174-529-3 • $16.95

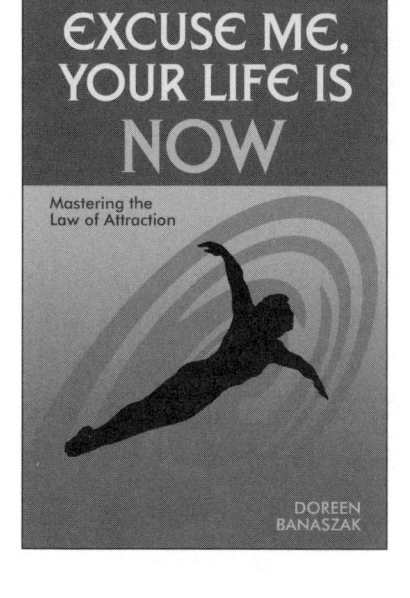

Excuse Me, Your Life Is Now
Mastering the Law of Attraction

Doreen Banaszak

Lynn Grabhorn's wildly popular book, *Excuse Me, Your Life Is Waiting,* offered four fundamental principles for attracting what we desire most in life. Now Doreen Banaszak has created a sequel that not only presents a convenient review of Grabhorn's four basic tenets—identifying what we don't want, naming what we do want, getting into the feeling of what we want and, finally, allowing what we want to flow into our lives—but also offers overwhelming evidence, including dozens of first-person accounts, that these principles really work!

Paperback • 208 pages • ISBN 978-1-57174-543-9 • $15.95
Available August 2007

Hampton Roads Publishing Company

. . . for the evolving human spirit

HAMPTON ROADS PUBLISHING COMPANY publishes books
on a variety of subjects, including metaphysics, spirituality,
health, visionary fiction, and other related topics.

For a copy of our latest trade catalog, call toll-free,
800-766-8009, or send your name and address to:

HAMPTON ROADS PUBLISHING COMPANY, INC.
1125 STONEY RIDGE ROAD • CHARLOTTESVILLE, VA 22902
e-mail: hrpc@hrpub.com • www.hrpub.com